Keeping Secrets and Telling Lies

Revealing the Truth About Disease and Self-Healing!

Dr. Robyn R. DeSautel
David Lloyd, B.M.E., GNM

2nd EDITION

Truth is the most powerful thing in the world, since even a single truth can outweigh an entire world of falsehoods.

- Paramahansa Yogananda

Contents

❧

Acknowledgements

I extend my heartfelt gratitude to Jill Bosonetto, my cherished best friend and editor, for her invaluable time, wisdom, and unwavering support throughout this journey.

To my remarkable children, Lexis and Jacey, your boundless joy and love have been my greatest blessings.

A special thank you goes to my parents, Donna Raus and Mark DeSautel, for the immeasurable gifts of love and support they have bestowed upon me.

Lastly, I am indebted to the countless authors and teachers whose profound insights have greatly enriched my understanding of truth.

-Dr. Robyn R. DeSautel

Introduction

❦

Over the past 150 years, there has been an alarming increase in diseases such as cancer, diabetes, Alzheimer's, and even conditions previously unknown, like autism and childhood cancer. This upsurge is neither explained by enhanced testing methods nor solely as a result of modern diagnostics. A mere half-century ago, these ailments were rare. Today, however, they touch nearly every family. What has precipitated this decline in global health, particularly in the United States?

We will reveal secrets vital to you and your family's well-being, delving into the deviation of health practices from their origins in the 1860s. During that era, the emphasis was on hygiene, sanitation, diet, and spirituality. However, these were soon overshadowed by an approach driven by diagnosis, pharmaceuticals, vaccinations, and, notably, enormous profits.

Louis Pasteur's questionable experiments led to mercury pills and vaccines being commonly prescribed. The founding of the American Medical Association (AMA) in 1847 further eroded natural health practices, branding proponents of herbs, hygiene, and nutrition as mere quacks, witch doctors, and snake oil salesmen. Big Pharma seized this opportunity to dominate the health industry, ruthlessly suppressing opposition.

This monopolistic control continues to this day, with Big Pharma manipulating fears around infectious diseases and cancer. The disinformation, censorship, and outright removal of those advocating alternative treatments are grievous wrongs, and they amount to crimes against humanity.

Our purpose is to expose this deception and shift the world into a new understanding, echoing Mahatma Gandhi's words: "An error does not become truth by reason of multiplied propagation, nor does truth become error because nobody sees it."

Sit back, get comfortable, and prepare to unearth well-kept secrets, the tragedy of Dr. Semmelweis, "Tricky" Louis, crazy Aaron the Rock Star, and his son Tiger. It's time to understand the events that have led to the decline in global health and what we can do to take back control. The time for truth is now.

> **"An error does not become truth by reason of multiplied propagation, nor does truth become error because nobody sees it." -Mahatma Gandhi**

CHAPTER 1

Do Germs Make Us Sick?

🍂

We have been repeatedly told that germs make us sick. Germs are everywhere; that is true. And, yes, germs can cause symptoms that make you feel sick. However, before we deep-dive into any of it, let's set the stage with a little story.

Imagine, if you would, you have a good friend who became a Rock Star. Let's call him Aaron. He traveled the world with his band, recording songs and singing at sold-out concerts. He has a multitude of fans, signs thousands of autographs, and makes millions of dollars every year. Aaron loves to wear outrageous and stylish clothing. It seemed as if the whole world was following him! People would dole out their money for anything he offered.

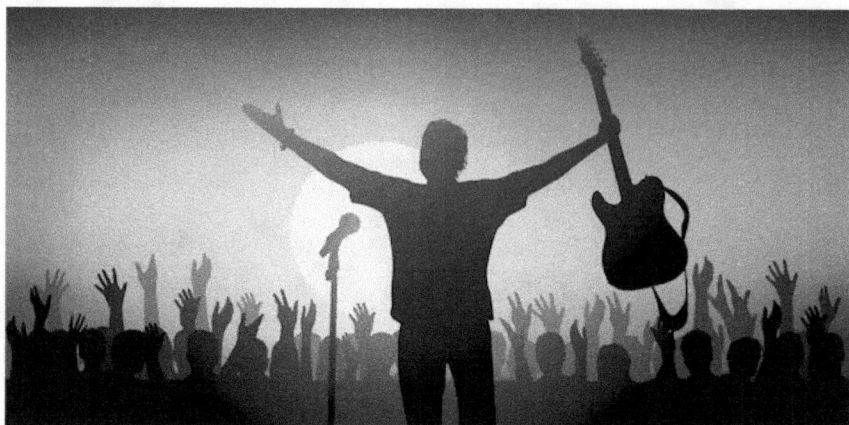

And then, as he aged, he was on his deathbed. You visit him in the hospital, and you see him lying destitute on his hospital bed. He has a hospital gown on, and you notice his trademark gold necklace with the gold microphone pendant. Then Aaron reveals something that astounds you. He can barely talk, but he extends his hand to you and slowly places his golden necklace in your palm. He wearily looks out the window and sheepishly says, "I have a confession...it's hard to admit, but...I want you to know something..."

You ask him, "What? What are you trying to say?"

He slowly tells you, "Well...I have to be honest with you...I never really sang any of my songs, I was only lip-syncing. I crave attention and adore it when people follow me and spend money at my concerts."

And you ask him in astonishment, "Who sang the songs?

He turns to you and answers, "It was Pierre, the lead backup singer. I only knew how to lip-sync."

How would you take that? What would you feel?

Back in 1895, something similar actually happened in the science community, and to this day, billions of lives have been adversely affected by it. There obviously weren't any Rock Stars back then, but there was a well-known scientist, Louis Pasteur, who had the same mindset throughout his career. He also made an *astonishing confession* about his life's work on his deathbed. Read the following quote:

"The germ is NOTHING, the terrain is everything."
- Louis Pasteur (deathbed confession)

The first secret is that germs are not the bad guys. They *don't* cause disease. They support you in your health! We'll repeat: germs don't cause your illness! Reread the first part of Pasteur's deathbed confession, "The germ is NOTHING." In the second half of Pasteur's quote, the word "terrain" is a French word referring to everything: land, soil, surfaces, tabletops, floors, part of the whole, etc. Terrain can also be considered as the overall health and condition of an individual. Reading "germs don't make us sick" right at the beginning of this book may be hard to take in, but hang in there with us and keep reading!

Why does this matter to you, your kids, and your family? Because our entire medical industry is built on the theory that germs (including viruses) cause disease. Germs have an *intrinsic purpose* in nature and biology and DO NOT cause disease. They may cause *symptoms,* yes, but not disease. Understanding the truth that germs don't make you sick will transform the way you live your life and understand your health.

We have found in our research before and after the events of COVID-19 that **a lot of misinformation is perpetuated and erased on the internet to keep the Germ Theory alive.** It's important to expand your references and look at multiple sources for history and information **because there are powerful entities that want to protect their financial agendas.**

We have been given so many drugs and vaccinations based on the theory that germs make us sick (Germ Theory), and many of these drugs and vaccines are harmful despite what we are told by misleading TV commercials and Big Pharma-backed advertisement campaigns. The list of ingredients that go into vaccines would make a Poison Control Center doctor go into a tizzy. A recent book called "*Turtles All the Way Down: Vaccine Science and Myth*" does a deep dive into researching safety studies of vaccines.[1] The PDF of the first chapter can be found online for free at: https://tinyurl.com/turtlesbookchap1eng

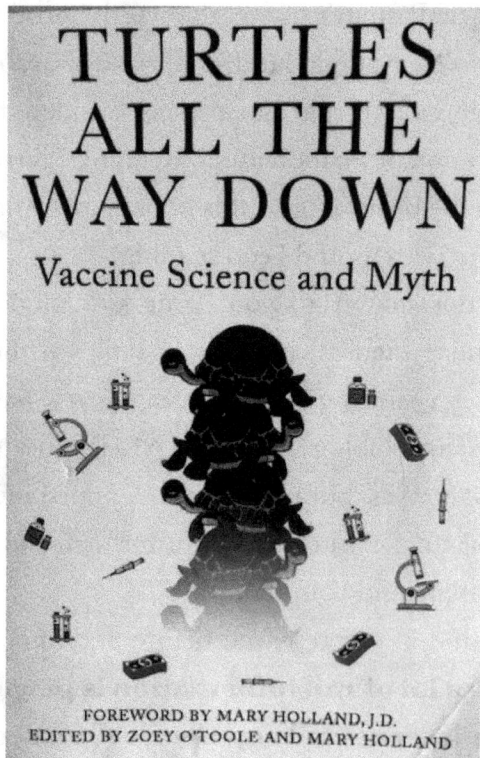

TURTLES ALL THE WAY DOWN
Vaccine Science and Myth

FOREWORD BY MARY HOLLAND, J.D.
EDITED BY ZOEY O'TOOLE AND MARY HOLLAND

One of the first questions people are quick to ask is, **"So, what is making us sick?"** Sickness is caused by toxins: physical, mental, emotional, and spiritual, and many times, it is triggered by a life event or shock.

- "Wrong habits of thinking and living breed all diseases."
- "Disease is an abnormal state of the body caused by an abnormal state of the mind."
- "Disease is caused in the physical body by the thoughts and emotions of the individual."
- "Disease often begins with the dis-ease of being out of harmony with oneself, one's surroundings, or the laws of God."
- "Disease comes from the mind, and disturbance starts from the heart. When the mind is calm and the heart is full of love, the body is healthy." [2]
- **Many times, what we label disease is triggered by a life event or shock.** After the perceived shock, the body does its best to attempt to *adapt* in the days after the isolating mental trauma. Sometimes, the trauma can be intense, and other times, it can be marginal. Everyone will have their unique response and adaptation depending on the intensity. One term we use for this adaptation is "tissue response." We will present more on this in the upcoming chapters, highlighting the discoveries of Dr. Hamer, MD (1935 - 2017) from Germany. It's also hypothesized that the shock affects our epigenomes, which control our genomes. More can be found on Ilsedora Laker's website at www. gnmonlineseminars.com.[3]

Why have we been so *ingrained* to believe that germs and viruses cause disease? Why did so many people die from the Coronavirus scare? Many doctors, scientists, and psychologists are now understanding more clearly what is happening in our bodies. They have found that a healthy and balanced relationship exists between germs and our bodies.

Hear us out! There is proof, and it all leads us back to Louis Pasteur.

There is evidence that Louis Pasteur, the father of the Germ Theory, propagated this modern medicine "truth" using falsified numbers, fraudulent experiments, and fictitious findings.[4] Yes, there is *actual proof* that his private notes and experiments were fraudulent.

Let's first look at what the Germ Theory is.

CHAPTER 2

What Is the Germ Theory All About Anyway?

❧

The Germ Theory states that *diseases are caused by an invasion of germs*. So, what is considered a germ?

A germ is a microorganism. What is a microorganism? A microorganism is a living organism that is too small to be seen with the naked eye. Microorganisms include bacteria, fungi, protozoa, and algae. A parasite is NOT a microorganism. Parasites *do* cause disease, but they are *not* germs. Examples of parasites are roundworms, malaria (plasmodium), lice, and fleas.

A virus is also NOT a microorganism and NOT a germ. A virus is a non-living DNA or RNA particle of a cell. Since it is non-living, it is *not* a microorganism (which is defined as living) and *not* a germ (although the internet will completely confuse these points to promote an agenda). Viruses cannot move or replicate on their own. They are often wrongly classified as germs, but it is important to know that they are non-living. It is well known that trillions of harmless viruses exist within every person. Every gallon of seawater has trillions of viruses. Viruses are very important in maintaining the balance and health of the ocean as well as our bodies.

Is the Germ Theory based on truth? Louis Pasteur, known as the Father of the Germ Theory, was paid by the French government to go against the scientists of the day. How do we know this is true? His private experiment notes were finally released by his grandson in 1964 after being hidden since Louis Pasteur had written them. A book was published in 1995 called *"The Private Science of Louis Pasteur"* by Gerald Geisen.[1] The book reveals all of Pasteur's notes and proves he falsified his experiment results. Most of his experiments were failures! Yet, he lied to the European people. How did he get away with it?

Before we get to all that, let us tell you a little bit about Louis Pasteur…

The Amazing Story of "TRICKY" LOUIS PASTEUR

Now listen closely…here's another little story. There once was a man named Louis Pasteur. Imagine Louis grew up wanting to be rich and famous. He wanted to be the Rock Star of his day! Sadly, he was not interested in truth, nor did he have much of a conscience. When Louis grew up, he decided to be a chemist. To make a long story short, starting in the 1860s, he was given a lot of money and fame by the French government to go against the common scientific beliefs of that time.

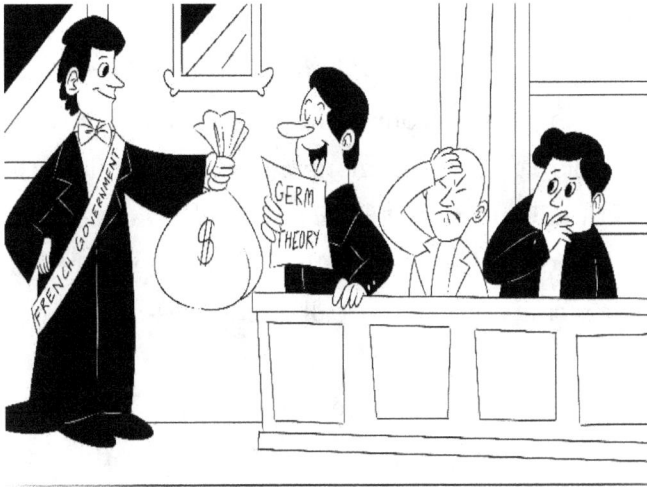

Stay with us here! Both the church and government wanted Louis Pasteur to "do research" in 1857 and prove that germs were not spontaneously created inside an organism but that they came from the environment. This was called the *Germ Theory*. It's easy to see how so many people bought into this pervasive, prevalent, but unproven theory. We are here to tell you the truth.

**"The bigger the lie, the more people will believe it."
Joseph Goebbels**

When the body is altered by toxins such as chemicals or stress, that's when germs are utilized to get the body back into harmony. Essentially, all DISEASE can be traced back to a DIS-EASE or a lack of ease. Rather, some STRESS that comes in a physical, mental, or spiritual form creates dis-ease. We have all eaten chemicals, parasites, or drugs that change our terrain. Most of us have dealt with the stress of overeating. But what about the stress that resulted from a fight or a constant worry about a loved one?

What about the stress that creates cancerous thoughts of anger, hatred, and resentment? What do these kinds of stresses do to our bodies? How do you think our bodies react and repair the changes?

This is where germs, commonly grouped as "microbes," come into the picture. Germs are *utilized in the body's healing process*, which has been altered by stress toxins. This is the reason WHY we see germs in the vicinity of what we call disease (dis-ease) in our bodies.

The assumption that germs are the enemy was based on the level of understanding our forefathers had. Unfortunately, that assumption is still perpetuated today! Imagine the world back in the 1800s: no internet, no air travel, no bullet trains, and no cell phones. The first phone was invented in 1876 by Alexander Graham Bell, and they were not widely used until the 1920s.

Go back in time even further. Think of how long it took humans to understand that the Earth IS NOT FLAT! It never has been. It took until the 17th Century for most people in the Asian part of the world to change their thinking about it![5] Millions of people in early Asia undoubtedly shook their heads and rolled their eyes whenever someone brought up the idea that the Earth is round. Some people still believe the Earth is flat!

We ask that you have an open mind *and* heart, and let's all emerge from the collective darkness of deception and walk into the light of truth. You may have an impulse to disregard everything you've read so far, but that just might be your Semmelweis Reflex. Keep reading!

CHAPTER 3

Who Is Dr. Semmelweis, You Ask?

❧

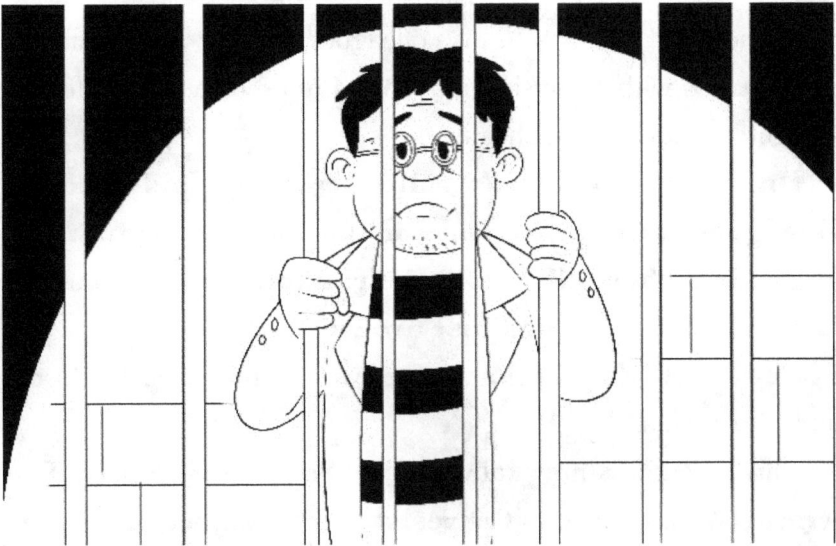

Before we continue, you need to know about the Semmelweis Reflex. We all tend to say, "That's ridiculous!" and roll our eyes and want to disregard information when it sounds like it's another conspiracy theory. We instinctively reject new ideas that sound contrary to what has always been accepted. This is where it is helpful to understand the Semmelweis Reflex.

Let us tell you the story of Dr. Ignaz Semmelweis. Dr. Ignaz Semmelweis was a Hungarian physician who discovered the importance of hygiene in 1847. He found that if doctors washed their hands after they did an autopsy and before they saw patients, many lives would be saved. Go figure! Now, we practice it in all our everyday situations, simply following our common sense. Dr. Semmelweis's studies on cleaning one's hands before delivering a baby showed that the practice of hygiene alone would reduce the death rate from 13% to less than 2%.

You would think he would be celebrated for his findings, but no! The opposite occurred. When Dr. Semmelweis presented his "revolutionary" findings to his colleagues, hoping they would be implemented with enthusiasm, he found himself locked up for his "dangerous" ideas about hygiene!

Dr. Semmelweis was called *crazy* by his medical colleagues *and imprisoned* in an insane asylum for suggesting they all wash their hands before seeing patients. Sadly, he died just two weeks later.

Get it? New ideas are not received well in the medical industry, public, or media.

This reaction is now known as the Semmelweis Reflex. **The Semmelweis Reflex is the resistance or rejection of new evidence or ideas that challenge established beliefs or practices.** It took over 100 years for doctors to finally accept Dr. Semmelweis's findings.

We explain this because *you* may need to overcome your own Semmelweis Reflex.

You might say, "Well, of course, Semmelweis was washing off germs," however, germs are everywhere. Germs aren't the bad guys. Now that we know Pasteur's actual experimental findings are nothing close to what was presented to the public, we can understand germs for their intrinsic purpose. Even Pasteur confessed that "*the germ is nothing.*" The cells in our bodies *naturally make* germs for a reason: to help us.

Semmelweis was washing away parasites and toxins found in dirt, grease, fecal matter, urine, chemicals, and bodily fluids like blood. These are the toxins that make the body *react* with antibodies, infections, and dis-ease. The body responds to these foreign intruders by producing GERMS. Our cells actually make germs for a purpose, which we will learn. Germs co-exist with us everywhere (inside and out), and when there is a toxic environment, they start their true work: decomposing, repairing tissue (acting as microsurgeons), and healing! We will cover more on this in the next chapter and throughout this book.

Let's clarify the difference between hygiene and sterilization. Hygiene is the cleansing of our environment. Sterilization is the killing of germs that are simply part of nature and harmlessly and helpfully co-exist with the whole. If someone must go into surgery after an accident, hygiene is always practiced. Sterilizing all the instruments is an *additional* step to have peace of mind from the perspective of the Germ Theory mentality we've all come to believe. However, germs are not the bad guys. Resist your Semmelweis Reflex!

Yes, we are happy that hospitals and clinics are hygienically cleansing their workplaces and instruments. Toxins and parasites are real and are the real villains of optimal health. They cause disease and death, and germs show up to repair or remove the damage.

Consider the scene of a fire and how the firemen rush in with their hoses and firetrucks to work tirelessly to put out the flames. You wouldn't blame the firemen for creating the fire just because you always see them at the scene. Germs are our firemen, but they've gotten a bad rap. They're at the scene of disease, but they didn't start the fire.

It is high time we embrace valid, proven, reproducible science that is not manipulated. We currently have a medical system that is based on scientific research, which can hardly be called science. When those who have the most money can pay for the propaganda that shapes our mindset and behavior, then it is high time we do our own research and form our own opinions.

CHAPTER 4

What Is the Purpose of Germs?

❦

"If I could live my life over again, I would devote it to proving that germs seek their natural habitat, diseased tissue – rather than being the cause of the diseased tissue." - Rudolf Virchow (known as "the father of modern pathology" and to his colleagues, the "Pope of medicine.")[6]

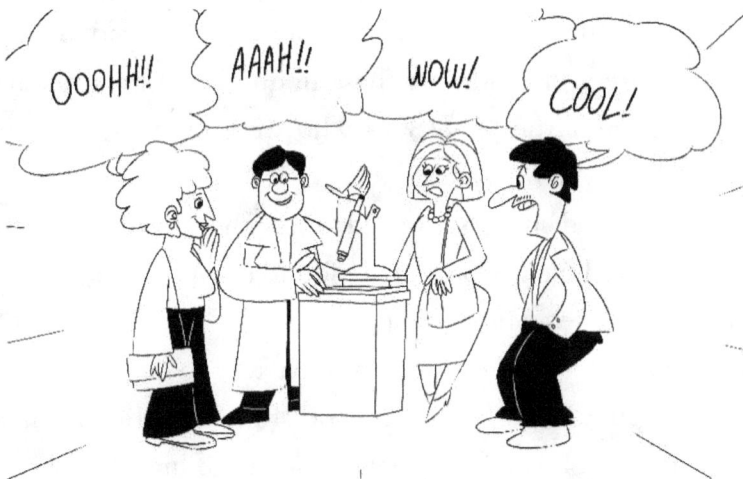

Antione Bechamp (Pierre Jacques Antione Bechamp, 1816-1908), a humble and brilliant scientist and professor, was known for many *reproducible* experiments to prove his Terrain Theory that tiny entities, called Microzymas, are present in all living organisms and in the surrounding environment.

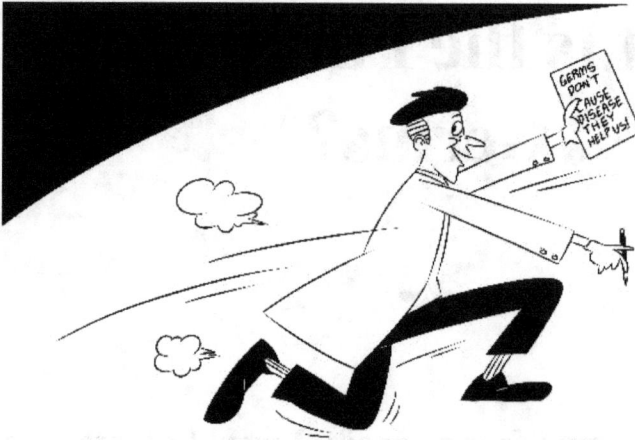

Bechamp's experiments proved that an organism would produce a germ spontaneously if it were in the presence of something toxic or if dead cells needed to be decomposed. Other scientists like Claude Bernard and Guenther Enderlein were also validating these findings. Let's call them the backup singers of the late 1800s who were overshadowed by a flamboyant lip-syncing lead singer.

Bechamp and others proved that the germs from our environment and the germs that are found in our bodies have their origin in this unseen Microzyma.

This diagram of the life cycle of a bacterium depicts how they are "born" spontaneously into somatids from the Microzyma and then further transform into other life forms. This all takes place within your own body. The cycle goes in either direction depending on whether your body is increasing in toxins and malnourished OR detoxing and nourishing.

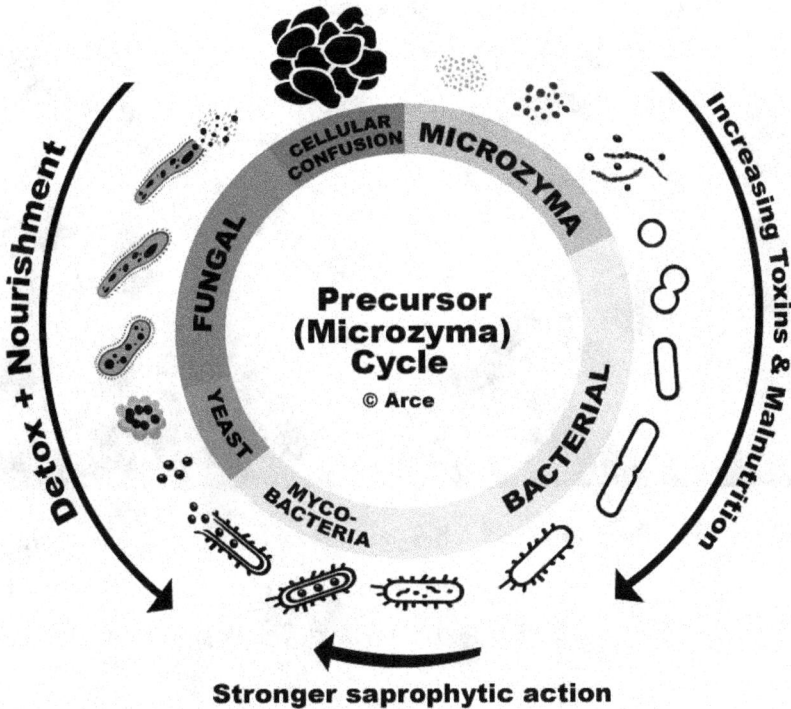

Image design by Dr Marizelle Arce[7]

Here's an excerpt from Rational Bacteriology by doctors Verner, Weint, and Watkins. *"Extensive studies of bacteria show definitely that there are no fixed species. A coccus can become a bacillus, a spirili, and vice versa. Streptococci and pneumococci interchange. All bacteria either acquire or lose virulence depending upon their environment. Bacteria change to molds and vice versa in response to adequate environmental stimuli. Furthermore, they can resolve into their smallest form, (somatids, sporatids and Microzyma)."*[8]

Even Nikola Tesla, the great inventor, knew this back in 1920 when he wrote, *"All perceptible matter comes from a primary substance, or tenuity beyond conception, filling all space, the akasha or* **luminiferous ether***, which is acted upon by the life-giving Prana or creative force, calling into existence in never-ending cycles all things and phenomena."* - Nikola Tesla

Electric Body, Electric Health by Eileen Day McKusick.[9]

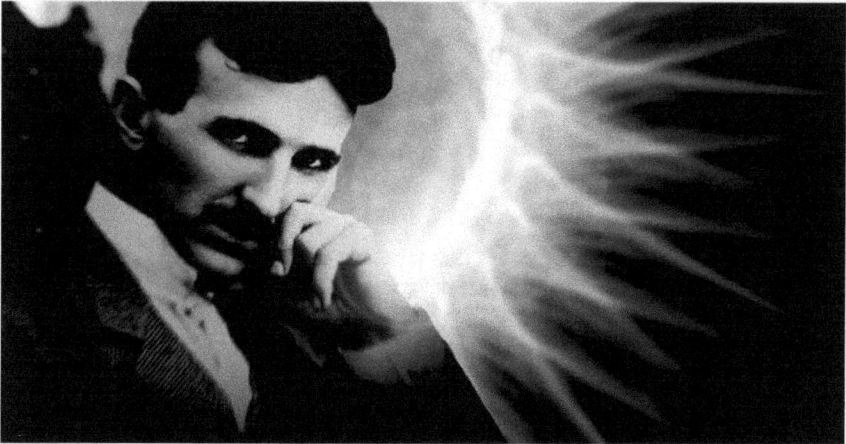

Bechamp proved that Microzymas are present everywhere because they're part of everyone and everything. From the Microzymas, he proved that bacteria develop by going through intermediate stages.

He also proved that on the death of an organ, its cells disappear, but the Microzymas remain, imperishable. He completely proved his theory that Microzymas were "in fact the primary anatomical elements of all living beings." As Carl Sagan, a famous astrophysicist, calls it, "star-stuff."

"The nitrogen in our DNA, the calcium in our teeth, the iron in our blood, the carbon in our apple pies were made in the interiors of collapsing stars. We are made of star stuff." - Carl Sagan (1934-1996) astrophysicist.

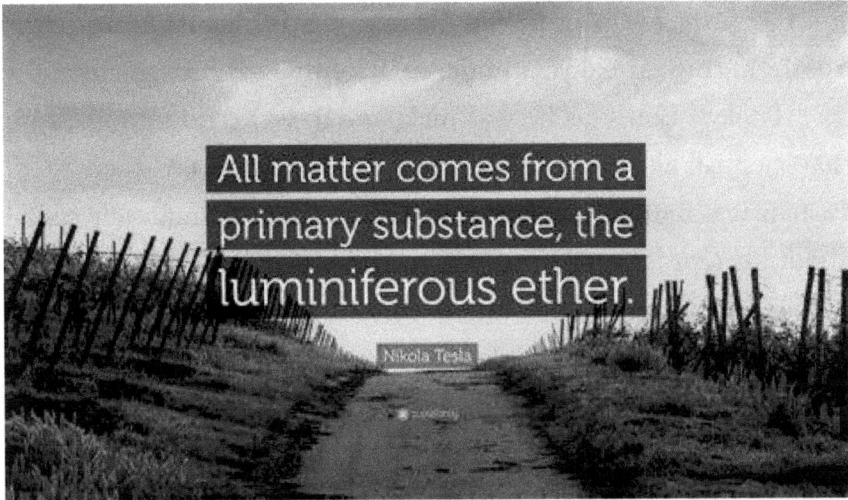

All matter comes from a primary substance, the luminiferous ether.

Nikola Tesla

Pearson wrote in 1942, **"*The bacteria found in man and animals do not cause disease.* They have the same function as those found in the soil or in sewage or elsewhere in nature: they are there to rebuild dead or diseased tissues or rework body wastes, and *it is well known that they will not or cannot attack healthy tissues.* They are as important and necessary to human life as those found elsewhere in nature and are in reality just as harmless if we live correctly, as Bechamp clearly showed."**[10]

So, just to be clear...Louis Pasteur had *no proof* of the Germ Theory (it should be called the germ invention), which says that germs cause disease. There is proof that Louis Pasteur falsified the results of his experiments.

Bechamp did reproducible experiments that proved that germs spontaneously develop from the Microzyma that is within and outside of you. Germs will seek out that which needs to be decomposed, removed, or repaired. **Just as the fireman shows up to put out the fire, the germs are present to help you heal!**

The *Germ Theory* promotes the man-made idea that life itself is a *WAR* and we are always under attack from airborne germs.

"Tricky" Louis (as he was nicknamed) was paid to make sure that scientists like Bechamp and their experiments were discredited. Pasteur was a great speaker and a convincing salesman. He spoke about his *personal* version of science *full of fraudulent results.* Helped by propaganda and government funding, he promoted his ideas far and wide (even though they were untrue).

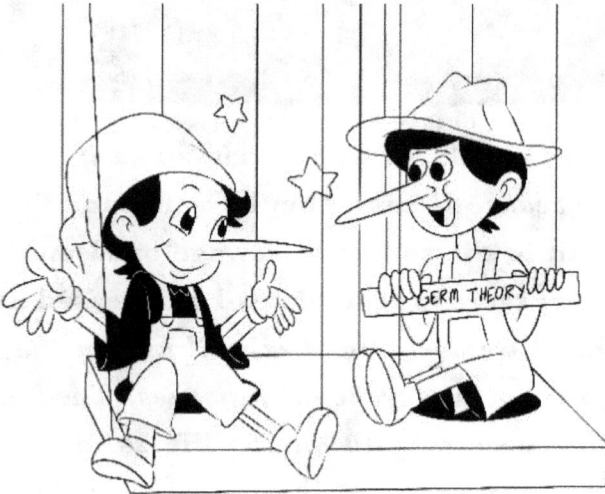

And what was he saying? Well, for starters, Louis Pasteur said that Bechamp's experiments were wrong. Pasteur claimed that germs were the cause of disease and that you could use *vaccinations* to protect people from these diseases. Although unbeknownst to the public, both his germ experiments and vaccination experiments failed. They could not be reproduced, and the true results were hidden.

So, Louis Pasteur, like our Aaron, the Rockstar, was just lip-syncing his way through the science. Other "Rockstars" like Bechamp, Bernard, and Enderlein could actually sing. Yet it was

Louis Pasteur who got all the fame, money, and glory by lying about his findings and by plagiarizing work from other scientists. To this day, he is still widely acclaimed as a brilliant scientist because the truth has remained hidden.

Two other comprehensive books that outline Pasteur's Germ Theory fraud are "***Bechamp or Pasteur? A Lost Chapter in the History of Biology***," By Ethel Hume **1919** and "***Pasteur: Plagiarist, Imposter; The Germ theory Exploded***" by R.B. Pearson **1942**.

Both books declare their intentions openly: that ***they wish to contribute to the undoing of a massive medical and scientific fraud.***[11]

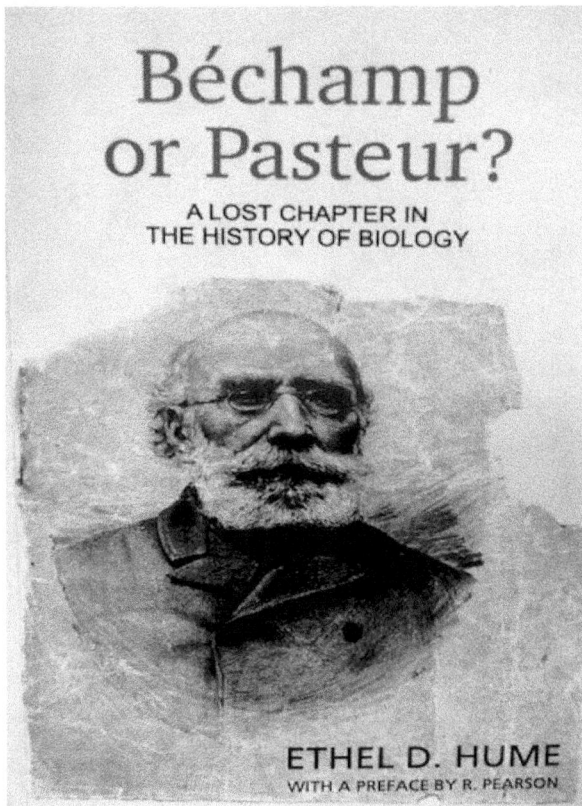

Béchamp or Pasteur?
A LOST CHAPTER IN THE HISTORY OF BIOLOGY

ETHEL D. HUME
WITH A PREFACE BY R. PEARSON

CHAPTER 5

How Did Those People Get Bloody Diarrhea?

Are you still with us? With every chapter, more lies are exposed, so keep reading!

Louis Pasteur became famous by saying that people were getting bloody diarrhea from a bacteria called listeria. He claimed that some cow's milk had been contaminated because the cows had the listeria bacteria, and now everyone who drank the milk was getting sick.

But get this! Listeria bacteria is found in HEALTHY cows. Also, listeria can be injected into healthy cows without causing any sickness to the cow or anyone else.

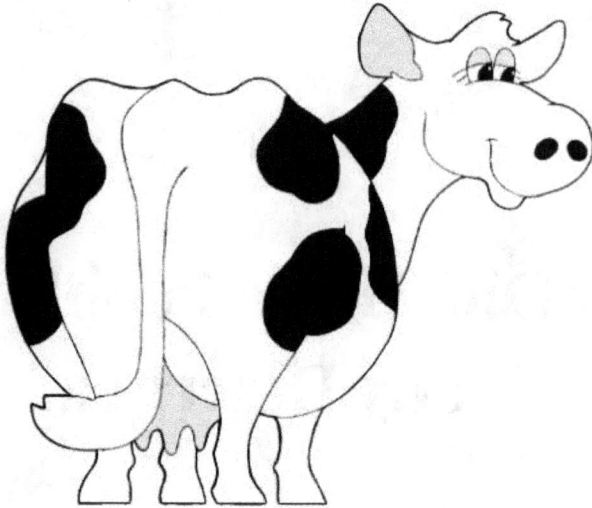

The truth of the matter is that listeria is *always* in a cow.

The cow was taking in toxins from drinking water and food that was contaminated, most likely from poor hygienic practices used in the barn to keep food and water clean. The cow's own milk was then contaminated. To be specific, *listeria bacteria was <u>breaking down</u> the cells harmed by the toxins in the cow's body, and it came out in the milk.* The listeria bacteria are like the fireman that came to put out the fire that was happening in the contaminated milk.

Experimentally, listeria was not the cause of the bloody diarrhea. This fact was hidden by Louis Pasteur's fraud. And thus began the war on bacteria, or at the very least, the **Germ Theory** began!

Here's an interesting excerpt from Dr. Tom Cowan, MD, and Sally Fallon Morell's great book, "*The Truth About Contagion*" (originally titled The Contagion Myth).[12]

THE

TRUTH

ABOUT

CONTAGION

Exploring Theories of How Disease Spreads

THOMAS S. COWAN, MD, and SALLY FALLON MORELL

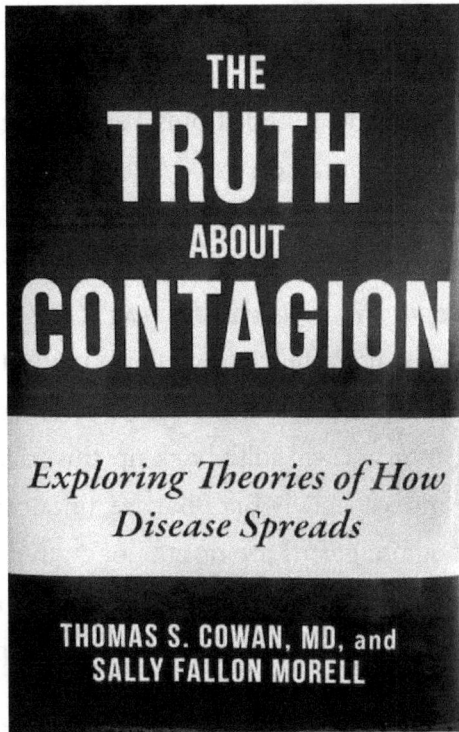

"Pasteur did this type of experiment for forty years. He found sick people, claimed to have isolated a bacterium, gave the 'pure culture' to animals—often by *injecting it into their brains*—and made them sick. He became the celebrity scientist of his time, feted by kings and prime ministers, and hailed as a great scientist. His work led to pasteurization, a technique responsible for destroying the integrity and health-giving properties of milk. His experiments ushered in germ theory of disease, and for over a Century this radical new theory has dominated not only the practice of Western medicine, but also our cultural and economic life."[13]

"Since Pasteur's day, *no one* has demonstrated experimentally the transmissibility of disease with pure cultures of bacteria or viruses."[14]

Read on to find out why no one else could reproduce these experiments!

Remember, on his deathbed, Louis Pasteur admitted that the whole effort to prove Contagion *was a failure*, leading to his famous deathbed confession: **"THE GERM IS NOTHING; the terrain is everything."** That concludes and proves *he MADE UP the findings that germs cause disease! He made it up!!*

Unfortunately, Louis Pasteur's fraud never made it to mainstream news. To this very day, we have the belief that germs make us sick. In fact, even the internet will fully back up this fraud because our whole medical world, especially Big Pharma, financially depends on it. So, we'll say it again: germs are not the bad guys!

Had anybody in power or with a voice in the media bothered to make sure that Louis Pasteur had notes or experiments that backed up what he was saying, we would not have the incredible health problems of today. Unfortunately, *Tricky Louis, as he was called, would not let any of his notes or experimental results be seen by any of his coworkers, colleagues, or family members.* He was very quick to discredit everyone else's work publicly, but he would not let anyone look at his own! His ego let him blatantly lie to the world.

Louis Pasteur, his whole life, would not let ANYONE read any of his notes or experiments ever! He made his family promise they would not release his notes even upon his death. Did you get that? He made his family promise not to release his private science notes even after he died!

It was well known that Louis *even* took his notes with him on vacation!! If they had airplanes back then, he would have been the secretive guy sitting in first class with the black briefcase handcuffed to his left wrist.

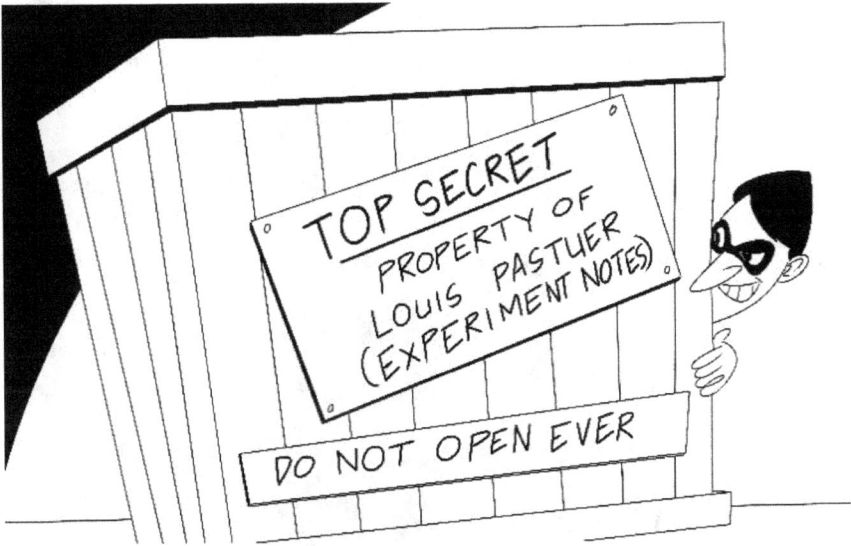

How do we know Louis Pasteur was making things up about his findings? Because Louis Pasteur's grandson, Louis Pasteur Vallery-Radot, must have had a true conscience. He finally released his grandfather's notebooks to the French National Library in 1964. The notes were published in 1995. Gerald Geisen researched and published Louis Pasteur's private notes and wrote a book about them. In his book, *"The Private Science of Louis Pasteur,"* by Gerald Geisen, Geisen confirmed what was known by scientists like Bechamp all along...*that Louis Pasteur was a fraud and a phony!*

In his private notes, Pasteur states he could not transfer disease with a pure culture of bacteria. He would sometimes grind up the brains of animals and inject the mix into *the brain* of another animal to "prove" Contagion. Or he would *add poisons* to his culture and then inject it to cause symptoms. Truly mad science! Pasteur spent a lifetime falsifying evidence to prove a hypothesis that science could never support.

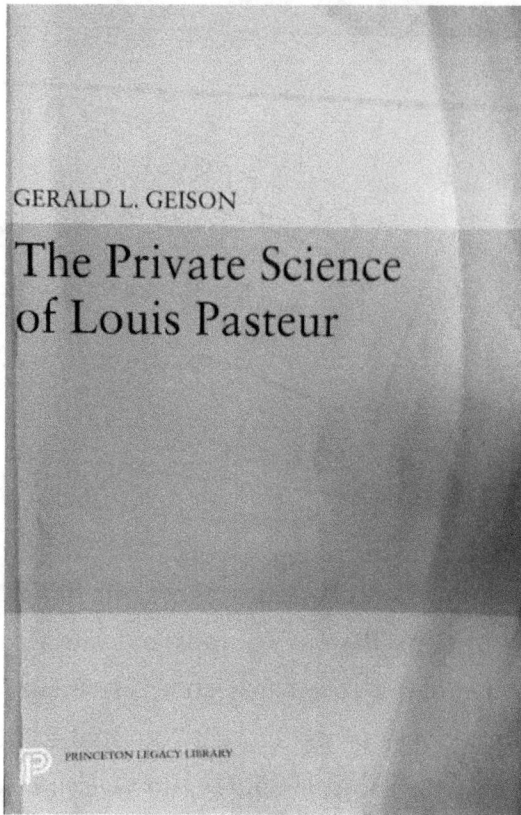

Geisen writes, "The conclusion is unavoidable**: Pasteur deliberately deceived the public**, especially those scientists most familiar with his published work." - *The Private Science of Louis Pasteur* by Geisen.[15]

The unfortunate truth is that since the late 1800s, fraudulent science has been promoted and paraded to the public, and the misinformation has kept us in the dark about our own power to heal from within. To this very day, Louis Pasteur is celebrated and written about as if he were a hero. And yet, *NOT ONE* of his experiments on Germ Theory or vaccines is *reproducible*. We will go into more detail about what was in his private notes in Chapter 9.

CHAPTER 6

What Does Florence Nightingale Say About the Germ Theory?

❧

Florence Nightingale, the most famous nurse in history, said, "There are no specific diseases: there are specific disease *conditions.*" She says, "Is it not living in continual mistake to look upon disease as we do now, as separate entities, which must exist, like cats and dogs, instead of looking upon them as conditions, like a dirty and clean condition, and just as much under our control." She says of smallpox, "I have seen with my own eyes and smelled with my own nose smallpox growing up in where it *could not* by any possibility have been *caught* but must have *begun.*"[16]

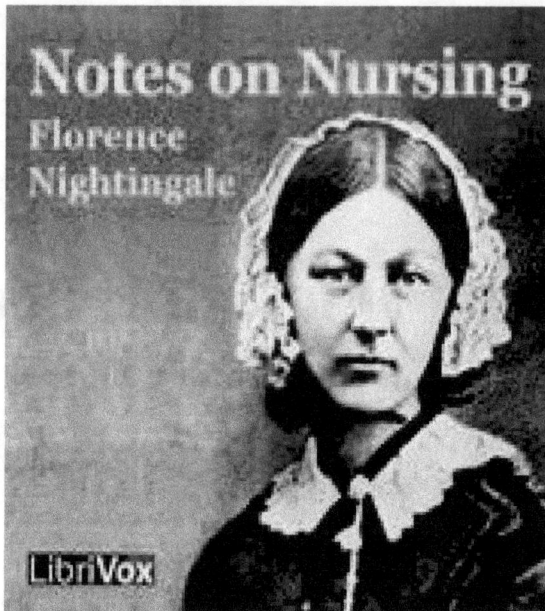

There is an overwhelming abundance of proof that the Germ Theory is a fraud and has been misleading us for over 150 years. We need only to look at the facts and scientific evidence to see the truth.

A good book to help you in your research is *"What Really Makes You Ill? Why Everything You Thought You Knew About Disease is Wrong"* by Dawn Lester and David Parker.[17] It has thousands of additional references beyond what we've listed in the back of this book, and it took ten years to write!

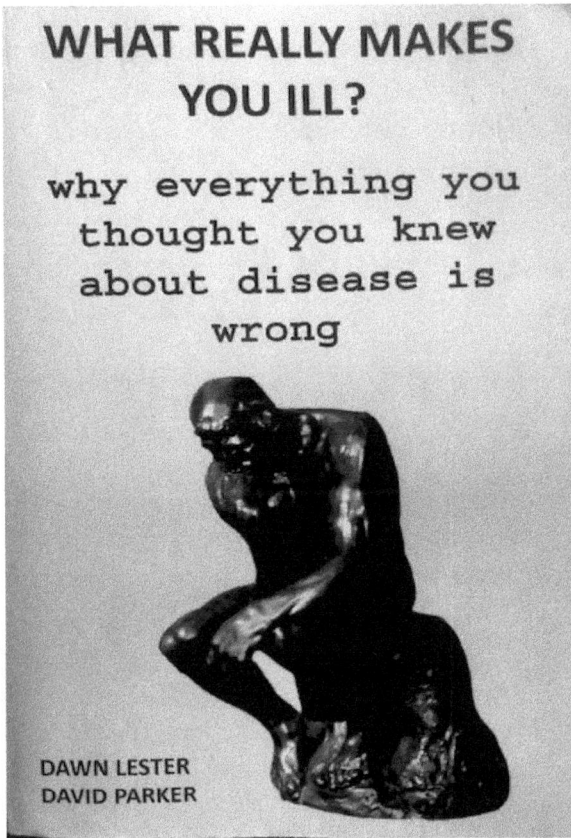

WHAT REALLY MAKES YOU ILL?

why everything you thought you knew about disease is wrong

DAWN LESTER
DAVID PARKER

We understand the information put forth in this book is an incredible departure from the mainstream understanding of health and wellness. But we only have to look around at the debilitating health conditions created by our modern-day systems, despite our advanced technology, to know that all that we've been told about sickness and disease may not be true.

CHAPTER 7

Has an Infectious Disease Ever Been Proven?

For a disease to be considered a disease, it needs to pass a test.

These notable offerings from science in the late 1800s are the famous "**Koch's postulates**." Robert Koch came up with four postulates, which are very commonly known by most scientists and doctors as the *"gold standard"* for diagnosing "infectious" bacterial disease. We all learned them in biology class.

Here they are, there are four:

1. The germ must be found in abundance in <u>all</u> cases suffering from the disease but <u>NOT</u> found in <u>healthy</u> organisms. (Remember listeria?)

2. The ***germ must be isolated*** from a diseased organism and grown in pure culture.

3. The isolated and cultured germ **should cause the original disease** when introduced into a healthy organism.

4. The isolated germs must be re-isolated from the now diseased organism that received the shot of isolated, cultured germs and identified as IDENTICAL to the original type of germ that was in the shot.[18]

The postulants make PERFECT sense. This is truly the only way to scientifically prove that a germ causes a disease. For example, Mary has whooping cough. All whooping cough germs must be found in every case for postulate one to be a diagnosable disease. Also, we should not find the whooping cough germ in a healthy person. For postulate two, we take the germ from Mary, isolate it, and grow it in a pure culture. If it cannot grow, it is not infectious. For postulate three, we take Mary's whooping cough germ, all isolated and cultured, and infect Paul with it. He must get whooping cough for it to be true. Lastly, for postulate four to be met, we have to take the germ from Paul and isolate it, and Paul's whooping cough germ must be IDENTICAL to Mary's.

This has never happened. No disease can pass this test, and yet it is the test a disease must pass to be considered a disease! Interesting right?

Not one disease **meets all four criteria**!!

We'll say it again...Koch's Postulates are considered the **"***gold standard***"** **for diagnosing a disease, and yet there is *no bacterial disease ever proven to meet the standards! Our firefighting germ may be at the scene of the fire. However, there are a lot of fraudulent scientists claiming that they have proof that the firefighter is the arsonist...***

Going back to the difference between bacteria and viruses, let's remember that bacteria are germs, but a virus (also claimed to be a bad guy causing sickness) is NOT a germ because it is not a microorganism and is not alive. A virus is one thousand times smaller than bacteria and is a non-living RNA or DNA particle that is part of the cell. A virus appears to cause disease because it, too, is one of the firefighters at the fire.

In 1937, Thomas Rivers came up with **Rivers' postulates.** Rivers' postulant addressed viruses, whereas Koch's gold standard only applied to bacterial infections. These also make PERFECT sense and are logical.

Back in Koch's day, scientists only had the microscope (invented in the 1600s), so they couldn't see viruses yet. Eventually, in 1931, the electron microscope was invented, and some scientists thought they were seeing the "culprit virus" that they had blamed so many problems on.

The Rivers' Postulates are as follows. Now, there are six:

1. The virus can be *isolated* from a diseased organism.
2. The virus can be *isolated* and made to grow in the cells of a new organism.
3. Proof of filterability—the virus can be separated from a medium that also contains bacteria.
4. The filtered virus will produce a comparable disease when the isolated virus is used to infect experimental animals.
5. The *virus can be re-isolated* from the infected experimental animal.
6. A specific immune response to the virus can be detected.[19]

So, did this help give researchers the proof they needed for blaming disease on bacteria or viruses? A big, fat NO! Nothing Further. NADA!

Researchers could not prove that a specific bacteria or virus causes ANY specific disease by using Rivers' Postulates either! Try your best to find one.

There are many *paid* fact-checkers who claim on the internet that the researchers have met Koch's or Rivers' postulates. It is doubtful that researchers even know what the postulates are when you read the procedures in the studies.

Dr. Tom Cowan, MD, states in the awesome book "*The Truth About Contagion*" (originally titled The Contagion Myth), "*No DISEASE attributed to bacteria or viruses has met all of Koch's postulates or all of Rivers' criteria. This is NOT because the postulates are incorrect or obsolete (in fact, they are entirely logical).*"[20] You may ask, "What? How can that be?" **BECAUSE GERMS DON'T CAUSE DISEASE!!** But Big Pharma and all the organizations chasing money will not let go of the Germ Theory fraud because it's *way too profitable.*

CHAPTER 8

Aaron the Rock Star's Cell Theory?

❧

"We need to change our paradigm and start BELIEVING that there is no war going on between our cells in our bodies." -Dr. Stefan Lanka[21]

Let's look at our cells in a new light. Our cells know how to function without our interference. We have been taught there needs to be some "extra" assistance for our cells to stay healthy. We have often been taught that our cells are under attack.

Picture a human cell as a bowl of trail mix. Cells are full of all kinds of small parts. Think of those small parts as the peanuts, dried fruit, chocolate chips, and raisins in all kinds of tasty flavors and colors in the trail mix. There is nothing wrong with the glass bowl full of trail mix sitting on your kitchen table. We all love to snack!

Our now infamous "Aaron the Rock Star" loved trail mix. He had bowls of trail mix in his house, his studio, his car, everywhere. His own son had the same fondness for eating trail mix, too. (What kid wouldn't!) One day, Aaron saw a big clump of raisins in the glass bottom of one of his trail mix bowls. He was puzzled how the raisins got stuck together. More oddly, he noticed raw brown sugar crystals in the wrinkled grooves of the raisins. After a few weeks of seeing those odd raisins in the bottom of the bowl, he convinced himself that the raisins should not clump together in trail mix. Something is wrong with raisins in trail mix.

Several weeks later, Aaron's son, Tiger, was on the sofa sulking. Aaron noticed his son was noticeably upset and angry. A kid a few years older than Tiger had stolen Tiger's favorite soccer ball at the park and was bragging it was his own. Aaron looked down at the table and saw four raisins left in that bowl of trail mix. He thought nothing of it at first. Maybe Tiger ate the clump of raisins along with some of the trail mix.

The next day, Tiger complained he was feeling sick to his stomach. Aaron thought his son *must* have eaten the clumped-up raisins! The raisins shouldn't be clumping in the trail mix. Something is wrong with raisins in trail mix. Aaron believed those raw brown sugar crystals were the suspicious culprits. He *knew* something wasn't right with raisins. Why are sugar crystals on the raisins? He started experiments to prove there must be something wrong with raw sugar crystals, especially the ones you see in the wrinkles of raisins. His curiosity started spinning!

He came up with the crazy idea that he could separate the smallest sugar crystals from the raisins and get more crystals to grow. He picked out three raisins with a sterilized spoon and placed them in another small, clean bowl. He was certain that he would find more raw sugar crystals within a few days if he added more dried raisins and let them sit overnight. He planned to feed the new crystals to his dog to see if his dog would get sick.

No matter how hard he tried, he couldn't separate the crystals from the raisins. With everything he did, there always remained a small bit of raisin along with each crystal. And if the raisin bit was too small, the crystals would disappear. However, he was so convinced he could prove the raw sugar crystals were making people and animals sick he told his bandmates, the backup singers, and his producer that raisins with raw sugar crystals in the wrinkles would make you feel queasy if you eat them.

Aaron was so charismatic that everyone believed he was onto something that would change the way people view raw sugar crystals. Aaron talked to his producer repeatedly and easily convinced his producer to give him weekly bonuses to further his experiments. Aaron kept his experiments going and took hundreds of notes, but he let no one see his notebook! At every new city where he played a concert, he would talk with people in high positions. He told everyone he had transferred bad sugar crystals from raisins in his lab experiments into other bowls of raisins and trail mix, and more bad sugar crystals appeared. In his loud-speaking voice, he proclaimed to everyone he hadn't had any failures. He said he then fed the new sugar crystals to his dog, and his dog acted differently. Aaron claimed he had successfully extracted raw sugar from raisins, and that is *precisely* what makes people and animals get sick. He told people the results prove, without a doubt, that raw brown sugar crystals are DANGEROUS!

Aaron was constantly trying to prove his point. After talking about it for so long, he heard other people agree with him that raw brown sugar crystals are attacking the cells inside of our stomachs! Without even questioning his work! After all, he must be a genius because he is... a rock star. Before too long, everyone was describing raw sugar crystals as "DANGEROUS and DEADLY."

Beginning with Louis Pasteur's delusion, this kind of deception is going on with modern, conventional medicine to this day. It is hard to guess how much Pasteur's mind was eating away at itself, knowing he was receiving large sums of government money, but we're sure his mind was spinning. Let's look at the quote he said on his deathbed one more time. Remember it?

"The germ is nothing, the terrain is everything."

In our combined metaphors, our Rock Star Aaron would have finally concluded on his deathbed, "The raw brown sugar crystals are nothing... the terrain is everything."

With Aaron, think of the glass bowl as a cell membrane, the peanuts as cell parts, the raisins as other cell parts, and the raw brown sugar crystals as harmless viruses all around the cell. In a sense, Pasteur was looking at raw brown sugar crystals in the wrinkles of raisins. All parts of a normal cell! Pasteur must have finally realized that he was looking at harmless particles as part of the whole. However, his mindset was based on the idea that if something is too small to see, and he could convince people he sees something no one else does, he can blame disease on what nobody sees! He was so set on convincing the world that germs were making us sick that he wouldn't admit he was wrong until right before he died.

CHAPTER 9

Where It All Shockingly Started

❧

We now know "Tricky" Louis was keeping a lot of secrets. From the pages of Louis Pasteur's private notes, we find several revealing differences from what he actually told the public.[22] He did hundreds of experiments on rabbits, dogs, cows, silkworms, and sheep.

In 1881, he did an anthrax vaccine experiment on a flock of 60 sheep in Pouilly-le-Fort, France. According to the private notes, Pasteur was deceptive about the vaccine he injected in the experiment. His notes show he used a serum that *another* scientist had originally come up with. The lackluster outcome ended with several puzzled farmers wondering why so many sheep died after being told Pasteur knew what he was doing.[23]

An even clearer example of Louis Pasteur's flawed "science" was recorded in "*Pasteur: Plagiarist, Imposter*," R.B. Pearson's book, where he relates an experiment done in Russia. He describes the use of Pasteur's anthrax vaccine, where 4,564 sheep were vaccinated, after which 3,696 sheep died! To this day, according to an article titled The Anthrax Vaccine Program: An Analysis of the CDC's Recommendations for Vaccine Use, "the anthrax vaccine was never proved to be safe and effective."[24]

In the fall of 1884, Pasteur made notes about a vaccine experiment with 26 dogs that resulted in a 38% death rate. The deaths were kept secret.[25]

In the spring of 1885, he did his rabies serum (vaccine) experiments on 40 dogs. The dogs received several shots spread apart day by day. Each shot was successively more potent. At the conclusion of his study, 20 of his dogs died![26]

That's 50% dead. HIS RABIES EXPERIMENTS WERE FAILURES! Yet, he hid it from the world!! We are where we are today with medical fraud based on Louis Pasteur's deception. Half of the dogs DIED, and he still lied to everyone by saying his rabies vaccines were a success!

Despite Louis Pasteur's failed dog experiment, he still flagrantly stated in his October 1885 paper:

"Fifty dogs of all ages and all races immune to rabies without a single failure."[27]

This was THE BIG LIE that started the vaccine industry. Did you notice how he exaggerated the number from the original 40 dogs up to 50?

Even more shocking, on June 22nd and 23rd, 1885, Pasteur and a doctor attended to an eleven-year-old girl. She had been bitten on the lip a full month before by her own puppy. The month passed, and a few days before Pasteur and the doctor saw her, she was complaining to her parents that she had severe headaches. This was on June 20th and 21st, 1885, according to Pasteur's secret

Keeping Secrets and Telling Lies | 45

notes. Naturally, they took her to see a doctor. After Pasteur and the little girl's doctor examined her at the Hospital of St. Denis on June 22nd, 1885, they *"declared"* she had rabies.

Pasteur and the doctor injected Pasteur's rabies serum in her two times, once on that first afternoon and another right at midnight. Another tragedy! She *died* the second day at 10:30 am.[28] It's all in Pasteur's private notes. Pasteur hadn't even finished his dog experiments! He injected her between the 2nd and 3rd group of dog experiments. That innocent little girl's name was Julianne-Antoinette Poughon, an unfortunate victim of medical fraud and ego. We mention her name in remembrance of her short life and all the other lives cut short since then because of one man's failed experimentations, which a corrupt system turned into *gospel truth*.

CHAPTER 10

What Did Other Scientists of Pasteur's Time Say About His Vaccines and Research?

❧

"In her essay, Dr. Morden refers to two medical practitioners who were contemporaries of Louis Pasteur but outspoken in their criticism of his work, as the following extracts demonstrate. The first extract refers to Dr. Bruette's exposure of the fraud of the rabies vaccine, "Dr. William A. Bruette, former assistant chief of the Bureau of Animal Industry in Washington, was also a contemporary of Pasteur and gave many proofs of Pasteur's incorrect findings. Dr. Bruette has proved, as a matter of fact, that the rabies vaccine is not only a fraud but harmful. He scorns the use of rabies vaccine and states that 'inoculation spreads disease.' He goes as far as to call the sale of rabies vaccine an out-and-out racket."

Although the current vaccines are different from those used in the 19th Century, they are all based on the same flawed theory.

"Dr. Matthew Woods, another contemporary of Pasteur, then a leading member of the Philadelphia Medical Society, wrote much on the subject of rabies. He stated that at the Philadelphia dog pound, where on an average more than 6.000 vagrant dogs are taken annually, and where the catchers and keepers are frequently bitten while handling them, not one case of hydrophobia (rabies) has occurred during its entire history of twenty-five years, in which time 150,000 dogs have been handled."

Dr. Morden cites a further quote from Dr. Woods, in which he suggests alternative causes for the symptoms that are often labeled as rabies as "fundamentally due to maltreatment or malnutrition or both."

In his book, Lionel Dole expands on the many problems associated with the use of the rabies vaccine, "Pasteur cannot be proved to have saved a single life with his vaccines, but it is quite certain that many people died from his treatment."

Dr. George Wilson MD, President of the British Medical Society, made the following statement in 1899 that was published in the British Medical Journal, "I accuse my profession of misleading the public, Pasteur's anti rabies vaccination is — I believe, and others with me — a piece of deception."

Although it is claimed that rabies is caused by a virus, the refutation of the germ theory demonstrates this to be an unfounded claim. There is, however, other evidence that also denies the viral cause of rabies, as explained by Hans Ruesch, a Swiss medical historian, who states in his book titled "*1000 Doctors (and many more) Against Vivisection*" (Vaccination) that "Medical students are taught that Pasteur solved the 'problem' of rabies in the last Century, thanks to experiments on dogs. They – and the public – are not told that neither he nor his successors have ever been able to identify the virus which is supposed to cause rabies."

In conclusion to her essay, Dr. Morden provides a summary of the mistaken idea about the existence of an "infectious disease" called rabies.

"Is rabies then a disease? Have we isolated a virus or germ? Is the 'Pasteur treatment' specific? Is rabies, in short, fact or fancy? I believe it is fancy, for I have handled so-called rabid animals and humans without benefit of Pasteur treatment and in *no case* has there been a death or any other symptoms of rabies. **I submit that rabies is non-existent and that the Pasteur treatment for rabies is worse than the disease, if it were a disease, WHICH IT IS NOT.**"[29]

Because of this "original sin" in science, modern medical institutions are continuously throwing darts in the form of sharp vaccination needles and barking up our trees with TV ads trying to convince us there is something wrong going on in our cells and bodies.

Our cells don't need any assistance other than food, vitamins, oxygen, and water to stay alive. Science has proven time and time again that the innate intelligence of the body has the ability to break down, remove, and/or repair cells. *CELLS COME AND GO; THEY KNOW EXACTLY WHAT THEY ARE DOING*! The dust on your dining room table comprises 20-50% dead skin cells. Did it hurt when the cells died? Did you even feel them fall off your skin? Every eight years, almost every cell in your body is a brand-new cell, with the exception of the nervous system and the female reproductive eggs! Some cells regenerate within 24 hours.

Modern medical institutions teach Germ Theory as if it were the Gospel. In doing so, it keeps us in fear of things they claim to see under their microscopes that "could" kill us. It's false! Again, two words: IT'S FALSE! True, honest science has proven it's false. Germs serve a purpose that is helpful. *Your body is extremely intelligent!* OUR CELLS KNOW *EXACTLY WHAT THEY ARE DOING.*

Many people say, "But what about pasteurization?" Aren't there harmful things in cow's milk? The only ones telling you that are the fearmongers. Common sense would beg the question, "How did my grandparents ever stay alive after drinking raw milk?" The only benefit of pasteurization is the SHELF LIFE of milk. That's it. That is a convenience for the dairy industry. We can refer you back to Chapter 5. The fearmongers will tell you that the bacterium in milk is harmful and will give you food poisoning, miscarriages, kidney failure, and the list goes on. The massive dairy industry is pleased when we fear drinking raw milk.

However, the data does not support this fear. The heating of milk kills every nutrient and enzyme in milk, making it virtually useless. Many bodies recognize pasteurized milk as a poison because it is no longer recognized as a food. Before pasteurization, milk allergies were unheard of. Now, they are commonplace.

Thanks to Louis Pasteur and "pasteurization," we have milk that doesn't spoil and fear of that which is a very nutritious food, "raw milk."

CHAPTER 11

Are Germs Helpful?

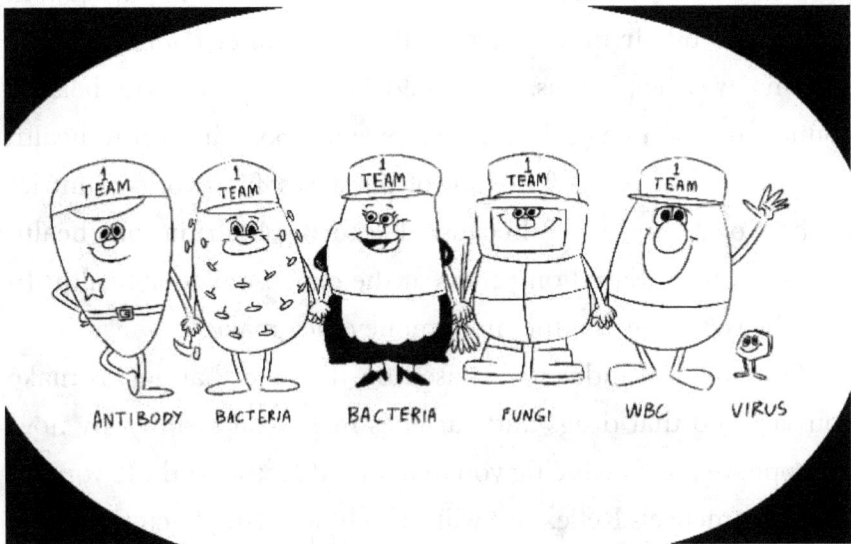

ANTIBODY BACTERIA BACTERIA FUNGI WBC VIRUS

"Unthinking **respect for authority is the greatest enemy of truth"** **- Albert Einstein.**

Over 150 years ago, the medical industry took off after using Louis Pasteur's false experiments and findings. They used propaganda to push the Germ Theory to make *trillions* of dollars on the sale of drugs and vaccines. They are still at it! How many prescription drug advertisements have you seen on TV within the last few days? It's modern-day propaganda. Big Pharma has media networks in the palm of its hand. It's a Catch-22 for the networks to either keep taking the advertisement money or find other ads and start honoring our health. Here's a suggestion: the next time you see a drug ad on TV, laugh and push the mute button.

Did you know that the United States and New Zealand are the *only* two countries in the world that allow drug advertisements on TV? No wonder we take 75% of all the prescription drugs produced in the world. We are only 5% of the world's population, but we are by far more drugged than any other country. If Big Pharma was helping us, we would be by far the most healthy country on the planet, but instead, we are 33rd in overall health compared to the rest. We are one of the sickest first-world countries in the world. And why? Because due to Big Pharma, our health care industry is based on profits at the expense of our health. In fact, the sicker we are, the more money they make.

Our medical industry is based on the idea that germs make you sick and that drugs and vaccines make you healthy. By now, we hope we are convincing you that it is NOT the truth. If you still have Semmelweis Reflex, we will learn how germs, bacteria, fungi, and viruses *work together* in our cells.

If you look at the dead cell tissue of a sick person under a microscope, you will *always* see germs *helping* clean up the area. And the cleanup and repair process *does* make you feel symptoms. "Think of it as a construction site, it's repairing itself." Caroline

Markolin, PhD. Learninggnm.com. It's important to realize **YOUR SYMPTOMS ARE NOT YOUR SICKNESS.**

*SYMPTOMS ARE YOUR ALERT THAT YOU ARE **HEALING** OR **NEED REPAIR** either spiritually, emotionally, mentally, physically or a combination of all four!* Yes, the body can heal and protect itself.

Bechamp was proving experimentally back in 1855 how germs come from Microzyma when the body needs to be cleaned up. The germs act like **house cleaners** produced from within the cells themselves and show up in the air when tissue is unhealthy and in need of removal or repair. Bacteria are electric generators when they're in the cell as mitochondria. When they come out of the cell, they act like maids or firemen. Viruses (more accurately called exosomes, see Chapter 15) are in the cell as electric particles that are helpful. And now we see, back in 2010, from the *atomic force microscope*, that they are released from the cell to act like sponges or cell phones. They are communication directors for your health! More about this in Chapter 15.

The immune system, which should actually be called the *support* system, is made up of antibodies, anaerobic and aerobic bacteria, fungi, white blood cells, and viruses.

All living organisms, from bacteria to your own body, are associations of these minute living electrical entities of Microzymas. Bechamp, with the help of Professor Estor, found microzymas everywhere, in both healthy and diseased tissues. He proved that the Microzymas were the basic units of life and were the builders of cells and tissues. "They also concluded that bacteria are an evolutionary form of Microzymas that occurs when a quantity of diseased tissues is broken up into its constituent elements."[30]

The germs of the air are merely Microzymas, or bacteria, set free when their former habitat was broken up. Bechamp proved with several reproducible experiments that microzymas were the living remains of plant and animal life. In the recent or distant past, they were the primary *anatomical element* of that plant or animal studied.

He proved that on the death of tissue, its cells disappear, but Microzymas still remain. As the Bible talks about how we go from dust to dust, the *dust* [30] of the Bible, the *star stuff* Carl Sagan writes about, and the *Microzymas* of Bechamp's experiments are *all the same thing*! We are starlight!

Quantum physicists now know that the smallest building blocks of life are made of light called photons. They make up everything. And we are all surrounded by a "luminiferous ether," which is the same thing as the Microzymas referred to by Bechamp.

Now, we hope this makes sense. We realize when all you've ever been trained to think is that germs are bad, it's hard to wrap your head around the fact that they help us! We're trained to think of bacteria as either good or bad and that all viruses and fungi are bad. But that isn't what is reproduced in *honest* science.

Remember, you've probably taken probiotics because it was recommended for your health at some point. And you've probably taken antibiotics because they were prescribed. So, the antibiotics killed bacteria, and the probiotics added it back. But what if the symptoms you were experiencing were caused by bacteria doing their job of removing the toxins? Your symptoms may have improved, but did you really get to the root problem of being toxic? What if the toxin stays in your body? What happens if you no longer have bacteria to remove it?

There are many scientists, such as Rudolf Virchow (1821-1902), known as "the Father of Pathology," who drank bacterial cultures of so-called "deadly" cholera in front of his students to prove that bacteria don't make you sick. He said, "If live bacteria are transmitted to another person, they don't develop the disease."

Dr. Max Pettenkofer, M.D., is also reported to have swallowed cultures of the supposedly "deadly" cholera in full view of a class of students on more than one occasion. Yet, it is reliably reported that he never came down with any illness. How brave, it takes the word "educating" to a new level!

The fact that *none* of Louis Pasteur's experiments could be reproduced should make you consider the reason he got his nickname "Tricky" Louis. He made a lot of money and received a lot of fame for creating and repeating disinformation. Remember, he was, in a sense, lip-syncing into a golden microphone...He was known for taking credit for the work of other scientists on more than one occasion.

And now we have Big Pharma: the medical industry, the med schools, the CDC, the WHO, NIH, NIAID, Research Institutes, universities, the infectious disease industry, virologists, charitable foundations, private investors, etc. (the list goes on and on) profiting *trillions* from this disinformation.

Remember, you are equipped with an electrical system that produces its own waste removal and repair system in the form of germs!

If you garden or observe nature, you realize this happens in the soil. If you saw a dead animal in the forest covered by fly larvae (which is one of nature's ways of decomposing a dead animal), you wouldn't say that the flies killed the deer.

If you saw a log decaying in the woods, you wouldn't blame the fungus. RIGHT!?!

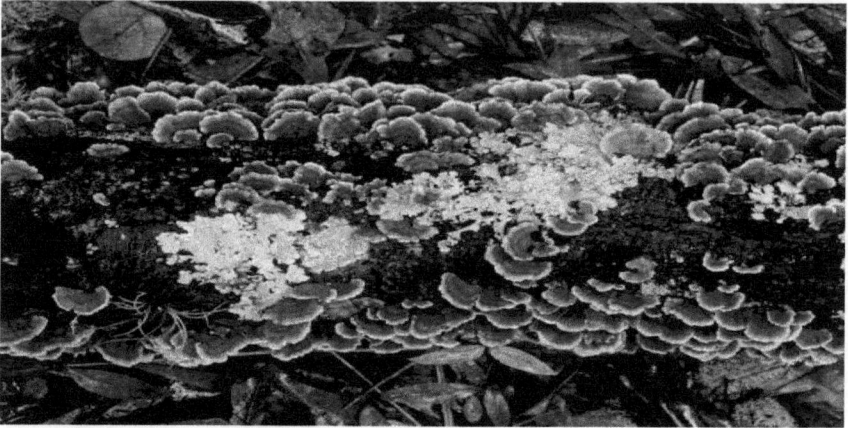

If you had a sealed loaf of bread and you saw spots of mold on the bread, you would know the bread was just getting too old and was being decomposed. And, although you may not like wasting money, you would understand that this is nature's way of breaking down the bread to decompose it.

So, even though the germ theory (which states germs cause disease) is disproven by science, and Pasteur's experiments were revealed to be fraudulent, the medical industry is *still* teaching us all that we need to be *AFRAID* that germs will make us sick or even *KILL* us!

Here's a quote worth repeating that started off Chapter 4, **"If I could live my life over again, I would devote it to *proving* that germs *seek* their natural habitat, diseased tissue — rather than being the *cause* of the diseased tissue."** - Rudolf Virchow (Father of Pathology).[31]

"The specific disease doctrine is the grand refuge of _weak, uncultured, unstable minds_, such as now rule in the _medical profession_." - Florence Nightingale[32]

"The war on germs would seem to be (financially) a worthwhile one, most likely due to a mixture of human superstition and greed. Out of this war was born _the oppressive medical cartel_ we are struggling with today. It's time we educate the people as to the truth and real purpose of these microbes and this fictional war. _**It's high time to say goodbye germ theory!**_**" -Dr. William Trebing, Goodbye Germ Theory**[33] (More in chapter 41).

That you or I could breathe and cause grandma to die is as likely as a robber could murder you by giving you a hug and a kiss. There is _no scientific proof_ that germs cause disease!

It's such a shocking revelation to realize you've been lied to, but we all have the choice to keep taking the red pill or the blue pill. To be clear, taking the blue pill is believing in the Germ Theory.

The advantage of waking up to the truth and taking the red pill is that you can truly realize your divine nature and power. Plus, your self-healing capacity!

Your body is filled with light! It is full of trillions of chemical reactions every second, and they are coming from the _electric_ source of light you are.

You are connected to the Divine Source, and all you need to do is improve your knowingness.

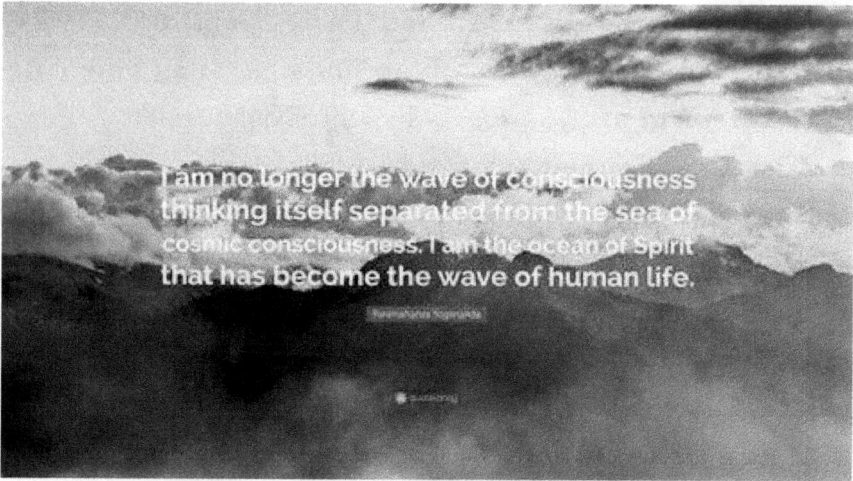

"I am no longer the wave of consciousness thinking itself separated from the sea of cosmic consciousness. I am the ocean of Spirit that has become the wave of human life."

"I am no longer the wave of consciousness thinking itself separated from the sea of cosmic consciousness. I am the ocean of Spirit that has become the wave of human life." - **Paramahansa Yogananda.**

So, now let's get a better understanding of what's going on with the bacteria, fungi, and viruses that are inside of you at this moment.

CHAPTER 12

Bacteria – Your House Cleaners and Repair Service!

❧

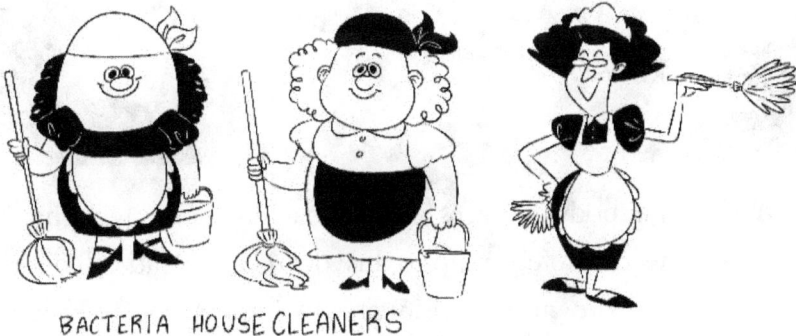

BACTERIA HOUSE CLEANERS

Like maids with sponges would be present to clean your house, picture bacteria working to clean up toxins and take out garbage.

You wouldn't blame the maid for the garbage! And you wouldn't want to kill them.

Bacteria are produced (out of the Microzymas) in the body when the body needs help cleaning up due to dead cells or repairs needed. They are present inside and outside your body. ***You have four times as many bacteria as you have cells (over 30 trillion).***

"It is widely accepted that mitochondria evolve from bacteria."[34]

Mitochondria are the energy-producing electric batteries of your cells and come from bacteria.

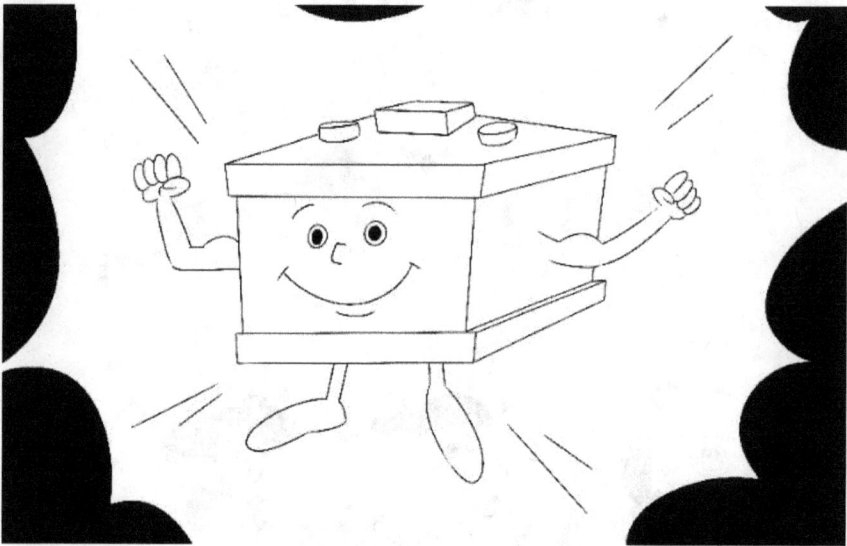

When your body requires certain bacteria, they will change into a form needed to clean up toxins, dead cells, dead cell debris, or repair. This is known as polymorphism. Staphylococcus bacteria are used in your skin and joints. Tuberculosis bacteria are used in your lungs and breast tissue. Streptococcus bacteria are used in your throat. These are just a few examples you might be familiar with, but there are billions more! We've all heard of probiotics and how good they are for you, especially if they're many different types of bacteria.

Does the following diagram look familiar? It's the one used in many science books explaining spontaneous generation and an older version of the diagram we showed earlier. Science refers to this depiction as polymorphism or pleomorphism. It's the cycle of our starlight somatids changing into spores, rods, bacteria, mycobacteria, yeast, and fungi and then back into somatids. Remember, the cycle goes in either direction depending on whether your body is increasing in toxins and malnourished **OR** detoxing and nourishing.

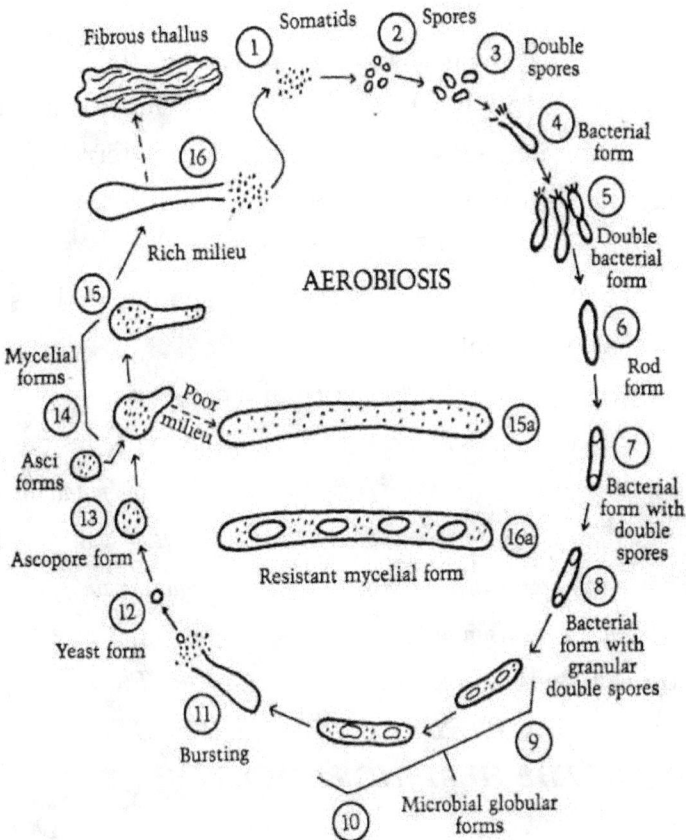

Here's an excerpt from Rational Bacteriology by doctors Verner, Weint, and Watkins. *"Extensive studies of bacteria show definitely that there are no fixed species. A coccus can become a bacillus, a spirili, and vice versa. Streptococci and pneumococci interchange. All bacteria either acquire or lose virulence depending upon their environment. Bacteria change to molds and vice versa in response to adequate environmental stimuli. Furthermore, they can resolve into their smallest form, (somatids, sporatids and Microzyma)."*[35]

We have all watched enough science fiction to imagine the shape-shifting character who can become whatever is needed at the moment. Imagine this amazing character in your body! This is your bacteria in action.

Every time you eat yogurt or drink kombucha, you are taking in LOTS of anaerobic bacteria that are just part of the fermentation process. GOOD and BAD BACTERIA are inaccurate names. They are misnomers. Bacteria are part of the terrain, part of everything. The terrain makes us think of a trail mix with jellybeans and wrinkled raisins! It ALL goes together.

Bacteria can also biodegrade many pollutants, such as heavy metals. It's been proven!

E. coli bacteria are regarded as a major cause of food poisoning, but it's also widely recognized that E. coli normally resides in the intestines of healthy people. *"The fact that they are found in healthy people who do not suffer from food poisoning is a situation that fails to meet Koch's First Postulate, which means that E. coli cannot be the cause of any disease including food poisoning!"* [36]

As the amazing book *"**Goodbye Germ Theory**"* puts it emphatically, ***"BACTERIA ACTUALLY BOOST IMMUNITY AND AID IN THE HEALING PROCESS!"*** [37]

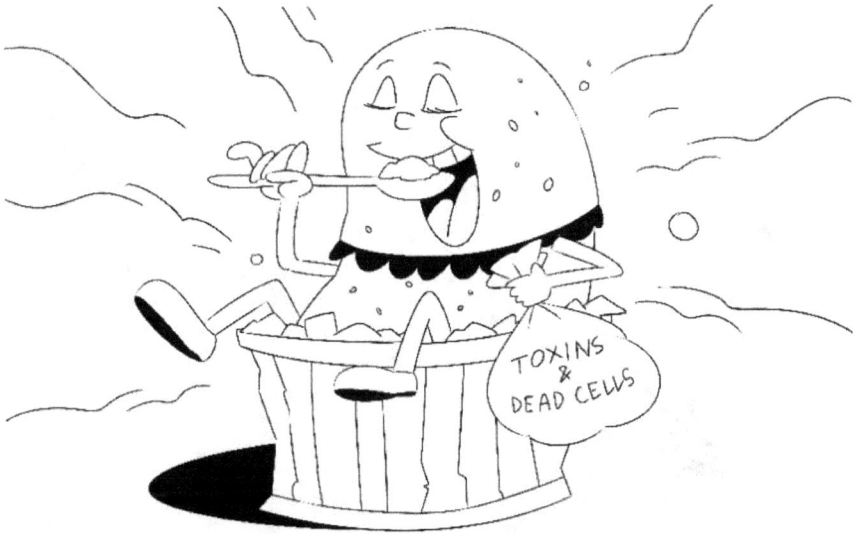

Bacteria will secrete enzymes to break down your damaged tissue. Waste products of bacteria excretions or bacterial "poop" cause some irritation which causes inflammation. **Inflammation is needed to dilate the blood vessels and bring more blood to the area to help remove the waste products. Yes, inflammation is part of the whole picture!**

Inflammation of this type assists your body by having more blood in an area that will help remove the damaged tissue. Bacteria need to do their work in a fluid, warm, and acidic environment. However, doctors call this an infection. You aren't being infected; you are being repaired. Again, that may sound completely backward. It goes against everything we've ever heard in our lives. Resist your Semmelweis Reflex!

CHAPTER 13

Is an Infection Bad?

When you have damaged or dead tissue due to toxins, bacteria or fungi will be produced to help you remove it from the body. Excretions of bacteria will often create symptoms called an infection. Do you see why any time you have an infection, bacteria will be present? The infection helps you remove dead tissue and toxins. Remember our analogy of the fireman being at the site of the fire? The firemen are the bacteria and viruses. They are there to help!

Florence Nightingale, the famous nurse, said, "True nursing *ignores* infection, except to prevent it. Cleanliness and fresh air from open windows, with unremitting attention to the patient, are the only defense a true nurse needs."[38]

These excretions of the bacteria (infection), which are often pus and fluid, will accelerate the removal of the waste products and speed up the healing.

If you use antibiotics, which kill the bacteria, you will stop or slow down the healing process from occurring. You will also damage the mitochondria in your cells made of bacteria. The symptoms might improve, but *then you still have the buildup of damaged tissue or toxins to remove.*

That buildup of damaged tissue will result in more "diseased" tissue, which can sometimes lead to a large overgrowth, which conventional medicine would mislabel "a tumor." During the body's healing phase, the so-called "tumor" will start to be broken down and removed from the body by bacteria. That is, by what bacteria are still left. The tumor will encapsulate if your body doesn't have enough bacteria due to the overuse of antibiotics!

Here's an example. If you are dealing with a chronic throat infection, most doctors will think it's *caused* by streptococcus bacteria. Yet streptococcus bacteria are there in your throat *all the time*! You will get treated with an antibiotic, which will kill your "bacterial maid service" of streptococcus bacteria on the tonsils. Doctors might assume the tonsils are far too full of garbage (dead cells or toxins) to heal on their own.

Your doctor may eventually say you need to have a tonsillectomy due to all the dead cell buildup. When we fall and scrape our knees, we soon get a dry, brown-colored scab. When dealing with the tonsils, the ugly-looking yellow patches are simply an *internal scab*. When babies get thrush, it's simply the inside of the mouth and tonsils scabbing over and repairing. The cells are healing.

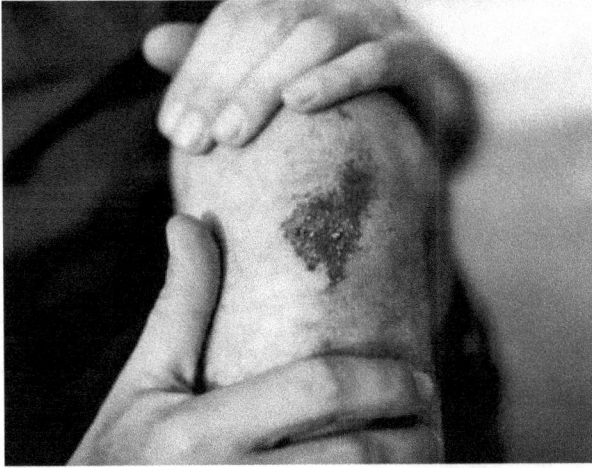

A much better plan would be to remove the stress or physical toxins that had caused the dilemma in the first place. Then, the bacteria would not need to clean up any of the dead cells, and your symptoms and scabs will go away for good. Take a minute to recall the last time you had a scab. Scabs are unpleasant to look at, but when has anyone seen a scab overgrow and take over a whole body and cause death?? Some "cancer" growths are simply *internal scabs* repairing cell overgrowth. At the end of the day, we are all going to have stress and be exposed to toxins, so the body will respond this way with symptoms if it's healthy. So, it's okay not to be stressed about the stress!

From Dr. William Trebing's 25 years of clinical research, he says, "When your body has reached a certain level of toxicity from your external environment, or more likely your dietary and drinking habits, what does the medical establishment say to do once they detect these bacterial healing agents? Wipe them out with antibiotics (translates: "against- life") and other types of drugs, and further turn your internal body fluids into a *toxic* soup."- Dr. Trebing [39]

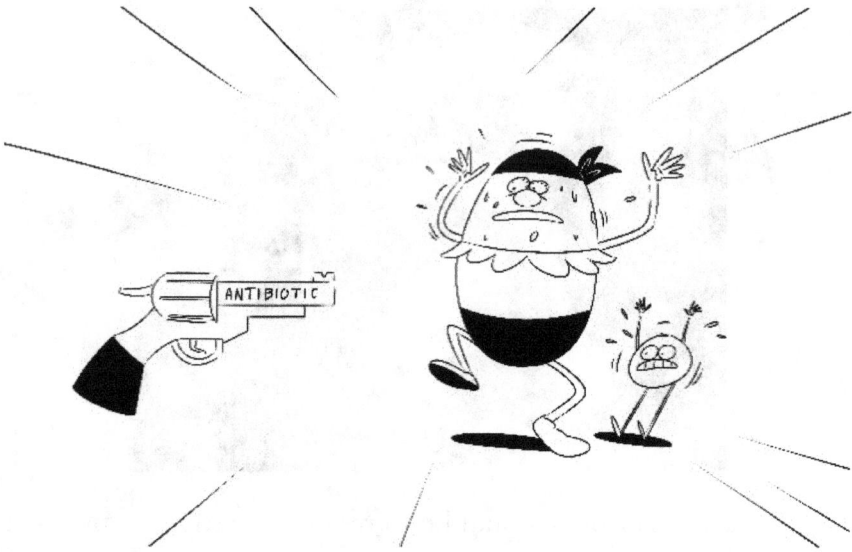

To be clear, you have been erroneously told that germs cause disease. The truth is every bacterium and virus you have been told causes disease can exist *harmlessly* inside you! Cholera, staphylococcus, tuberculosis, Ebola, streptococcus, and E. coli are all in your body, ready to be made from the microzymas when you need them. When you are healthy, you don't need as many bacteria or germs for cleanup or repair.

When you are sick or toxic, germs will show up (because they are produced by your body out of the Microzyma) and cause symptoms of inflammation or infection, which are there to clean up the actual problem.

The problem isn't the infection. The infection results from toxins. Focus on the toxins! Do you have any emotional, spiritual, mental, or physical toxins that are active or present? Clean up the toxins and resolve any life conflicts to help the germs do their job, and your infectious symptoms will go away.

Just to be clear, sometimes medical intervention *is needed*. Sometimes, you need intervention to *slow down* the infectious repair if the symptoms are too painful or life-threatening. There are circumstances in which a person's body is too full of toxins to repair all at once. Our common sense would hopefully help us know when medical intervention is needed in certain situations.

CHAPTER 14

What About Fungi?

❖

Fungi also come from Microzymas within the body. If you look back at the life cycle of bacteria in the diagram in Chapter 12, you'll see it involves fungi. Fungi are needed for the cleanup or repair of many cancers.

Fungi are like house cleaners or repairmen with hazmat suits. In other words, if an area of your body has been *toxic for a longer time*, it may produce fungi to help break down the dead cells. This process of one bacterium changing to different bacteria or fungi is called polymorphism or pleomorphism. It is how one disease can turn into another disease, but it's all part of the same process.

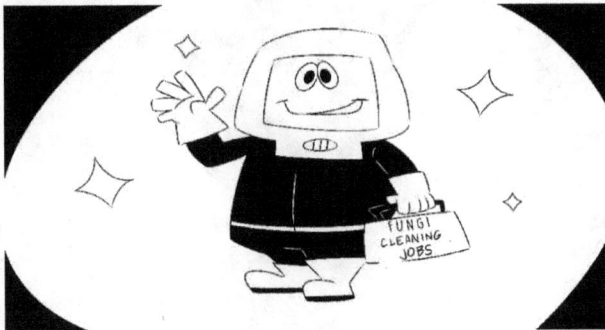

Fungi like candida remove certain types of cancer like breast cancer, pancreatic cancer, lung cancer, and colon cancer, along with other cellular debris in the healing phase. Remember the picture of the dead log with all the fungi growing on it? It's in its breakdown phase! It's important when thinking about any infection to get the root cause of the stress (mental, physical, spiritual, or emotional) toxins.

C H A P T E R   1 5

So, What's the Truth About Viruses?

❧

So, what actually is a virus? **This is where it gets really exciting!** Well, we hope exciting isn't an overstatement for you, but at least you'll *see the truth of how God made you so AMAZING!*

You have these little, teeny tiny particles called viruses or, more recently called, "exosomes" that are made in all your cells to be released when the cell is threatened or needs repair. When released, they act like electric sponges and cell phones. If there is something toxic around the cell, the cell will release these particles so the cell can be protected. These little particles also communicate with all the other cells of the body once they've been released. They communicate there is something harmful present and that it is time to get to work! To simplify this, picture the big orange traffic barrels and cones we have a love-hate relationship with when we're driving through construction zones. In a sense, exosomes put miniature orange traffic barrels and cones up inside our bodies!

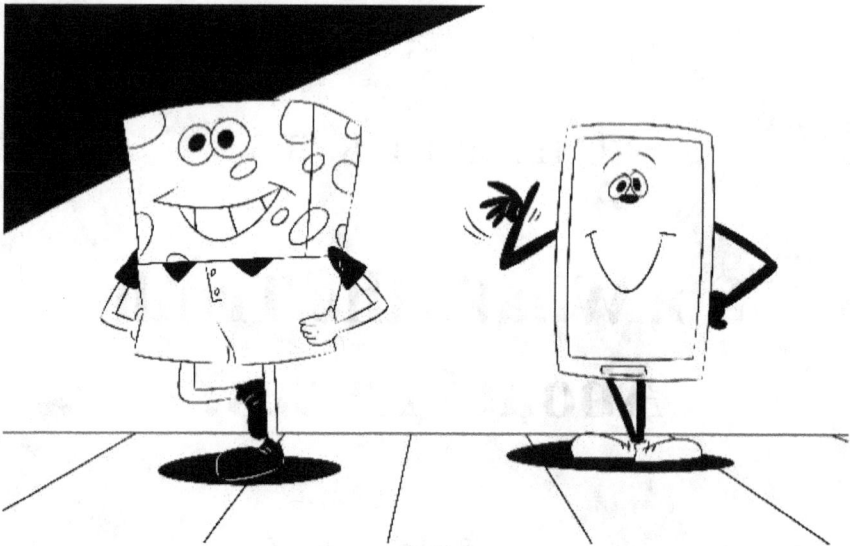

Viruses are about 20-400 nm (10x smaller than bacteria). They are the most abundant biological entities on the planet. There are 380,000,000,000,000 (380 trillion) viruses *in you*. Good thing they AREN'T actually BAD!

Viruses are either an mRNA or a DNA strand, and they are surrounded by a protein shell. What does that mean? It means they exist within the cell as nano-particulates. All scientists have agreed that viruses are non-living. Some scientists say it's only cellular debris. However, scientists who look can see that they are very geometrically shaped. *They are far too beautifully shaped to be garbage.*

Most scientists have been claiming that viruses cause disease by invading the cell, multiplying, and "infecting" it. This unfortunate *reversal* of the truth has created an untold loss of health and life. Because viruses don't ever "invade" or infect a cell! They help you!!

Consider the virus to be the most numerous form on Earth. As we already mentioned, viruses are actually helpful in sustaining the biological processes on the planet rather than infecting everyone and everything.

There are about 1 million viruses that would fit on a pencil tip. Your body is *filled* with them. There are over 10 *billion* species of viruses in one gallon of seawater. *If* they were truly deadly or dangerous, you really shouldn't go in the ocean water! And, if Big Pharma or the CDC could convince you that seawater was dangerous so they could sell you an anti-viral body condom, they would! At the very least, they would *own the patent*. But viruses aren't deadly or dangerous. **They simply help you when you need it.** God made you amazing!! Once again, they come out to help you remove toxins, repair and have intracellular communication.

According to James Hildreth, MD, President and Chief Executive Officer of Maharry Medical College, a former professor at Johns Hopkins and HIV researcher, "The *virus is fully an* **exosome** *in every sense of the word.*" **Exosomes are released when the cells are *in the presence* of:**

- Toxic substances
- Stress (fear)
- Ionizing radiation
- Injury
- Electro-magnetic frequencies (EMF)

Exosomes/viruses are released to help the body to remove these toxins and to protect the cell!

In 2010, the Atomic Force Microscope was used to view *live* cells in relation to viruses (exosomes) by Shivani Sharma, who has a Ph.D. in Biomedical Engineering. She was observing how these particles come out of the cells to *aid* the cell. And the research shows that exosomes and viruses are the exact same thing!

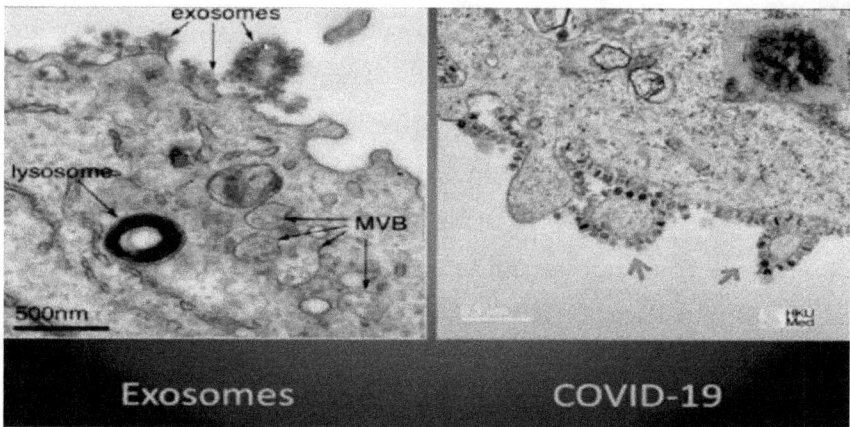

"*Exosomes (viruses) act much like a sponge preventing the toxins for a time from attacking the cell while toxins that are not corralled are left to burrow through cell membranes,*" says another study by a co-senior investigator, Ken Caldwell, PhD. [43]

Another researcher, Dr. Ian Dixon, writes, "The more research that is done into exosome function, the more we discover the pivotal role they play in development, in maintaining health, in the processes of aging and in disease." He also states, "Exosomes have been shown to be key mediators of cell-to-cell communication, delivering a distinct cargo of lipids, proteins, and nucleic acids that reflects their cell of origin. Exosomes released by regenerative cells such as stem cells, for example, are potent drivers of healing and repair."[40]

They can see these exosomes (viruses) are actually surrounding the toxins and communicating with other cells to alert the cells to toxins.

Once you realize the research that viruses are coming out of your cells to help you and that there is NO research showing the virus causes any disease (including the coronavirus), you will have a mind that is at ease! Viruses and germs are present all the time and only get released when you have some kind of toxin present. They get released NOT to make you sick but to help you get *healthy*!

CHAPTER 16

What About Contagion? It Seems Like People Catch a Cold or the Flu

In our 30 years of clinical practice, we never worried about "catching" a cold or the flu. We've had well over 270,000 patient visits and always thought that if our immune systems stayed healthy, it wouldn't matter what was going around. And we rarely got sick. After doing research, we realized it was NOT about our immune systems and germs.

There are never any disease-causing germs flying around. Yes, there are toxins that make you ill. But there are *real* studies that have proven you *can't* get sick by "catching anything" or making anyone else sick, for that matter! And there is NO study you will find that proves contagion if you do your research, which we highly recommend. Here are some known studies on contagion from the series "The End of Covid". These are from the section

"The Narrative (Act 2)", Video 11, "*The Proof of Contagion*" by Dawn Lester, Mike Stone & Jacob Diaz.[41]

FLU RELATED EXPERIMENTS AND THEIR FINDINGS

1906: Davis et al. attempted to infect one healthy person with Influenza by injecting them with secretions from an individual suffering from Influenza. This person did not become ill.

1916: Charles Fort – Dr Arthur W. Waite, who was an embarrassment to medical science, conducted his own private devious experiment on his father-in-law. In his bacteriological laboratory, he had billions of germs. Waite planned to kill his father-in-law, John E. Peck, 435 Riverside Drive, New York City. He fed the old man germs of Diphtheria but got no results. He induced Peck to use a nasal spray, in which he had planted colonies of the Tuberculosis bacteria. The old man didn't even develop a cough. He fed Peck calomel, a toxic mercury concoction, to weaken his resistance. He turned loose hordes of germs from typhoid and then influenza. In desperation, he lost all standing in the annals of distinctive crimes and went common or used arsenic. The old-fashioned method was a success. Peck finally died of arsenic poisoning. One's impression is that, if anything, diets and inhalations of germs may be healthful.

1917: Dold et al. injected 40 healthy people with nasal secretions taken from one ill person, and 0/40 [none of the] healthy people became ill.

1918: Selter et al. took mucous secretions from 5 people and sprayed them into the noses and mouths of 2 healthy people. 0/2 became ill.

1918: Nuzum et al. conducted two separate experiments trying to infect seven healthy people by spraying mucous secretions taken from one ill person (who supposedly had the "contagious" Spanish Flu) into their nasal passages, and 0/7 became ill.

1919: In 1919, Wahl et al. conducted three separate experiments to infect six healthy men with Influenza (Spanish Flu) by exposing them to mucous secretions and lung tissue from sick people. 0/6 men contracted Influenza in any of the three studies.

Also, in 1919 Yamanouchi et al. sprayed infected mucous into the noses and throats of healthy men. 0/14 became ill.

In March of 1919, Rosenau & Keegan conducted nine separate experiments in a group of 49 healthy men to prove contagion from the Spanish Flu. In all nine experiments, 0/49 men became sick after being exposed to sick people or the bodily fluids of sick people.

In November of 1919, Rosenau et al. conducted eight separate experiments in a group of 62 men, trying to prove that Influenza is contagious and causes disease. In all eight experiments, 0/62 men became sick.

McCoy et al. undertook a set of 8 experiments in December of 1919 on 50 men to try and prove contagion. Once again, all eight experiments failed to prove people with Influenza or their bodily fluids cause illness; 0/50 men became sick.

1920: Bloomfield et al. exposed healthy men to mucous secretions taken from sick people; 0/14 became ill.

1930: In 1930, Dochez et al. attempted to infect a group of men experimentally with the common cold. The authors stated in their results something that is nothing short of amazing. They stated that it was apparent very early that there was one individual who was unreliable, and from the start, it was impossible to keep him in the dark regarding their procedure. He had inconspicuous symptoms after his test injection of sterile broth and no more striking results from the cold filtrate until an assistant, on the second day after injection, inadvertently referred to this failure to contract a cold. That evening and night, the subject reported severe symptoms, including sneezing, cough, sore throat, and stuffiness in the nose. The next morning, he was told that he had been misinformed in regard to the nature of the filtrate, and his symptoms subsided within the hour. It is important to note that there was an entire absence of objective pathological changes. This brings up the importance of the "expectation effect," which we will explain in the next chapter.

1937: Burnet & Lush conducted an experiment exposing 200 healthy people to bodily secretions from people infected with Influenza. 0/200 became sick.

1940: Francis et al. exposed healthy men to the mucous taken from an infected person, and 0/11 became ill.

1940: Burnet and Foley tried to experimentally infect 15 university students with Influenza. The authors concluded their experiment was a failure. 0/15 became ill.

2003: Bridges et al. reviewed Influenza transmissions and found "no human experimental studies published in the English language literature delineating person-to-person transmission of Influenza."

Similar studies by Beare et al. on other H1N1 viruses found that 46 of 55 directly inoculated volunteers failed to develop symptoms.

OTHER RELATED EXPERIMENTS AND THEIR FINDINGS

1923: Ludvig Hektoen, MD, published a paper in JAMA titled "The History of Experimental Scarlet Fever in Man." In this paper, Hektoen reviewed the human experiments attempting to transmit Scarlet Fever between sick people and healthy people. He concluded: "This brief review of the recorded attempts to produce Scarlet Fever experimentally in man reveals that it is exceedingly doubtful whether a single positive case has been obtained. In view of the ease with which Scarlet Fever appears to be transmitted under natural conditions, the failure of the efforts at experimental transmission is a perplexing puzzle that awaits solution."

Our answer to the "perplexing puzzle" Hektoen, MD refers to comes from the understanding that toxins (including fear) cause dis-ease. Again, this is the "expectation effect," which we will explain in the next chapter.

1962: In 1962, an experiment was conducted to try to infect the skin of healthy participants with the fungus Candida albicans. Everything was done to infect the skin, including abrading or scarifying the skin and then applying a thick layer of the fungus. In no instance did an infection occur. The authors concluded, "If the site was not covered, even if massive numbers of organisms were applied daily for 7 days, infection didn't occur. Mere contamination of the skin with this organism is not sufficient to produce infection under ordinary conditions."

This experiment is touted as proof that Candida causes skin infections. What do you think?

1994: On December 7, at Hollywood Roosevelt Hotel, Greensboro, N.C., Dr. Willner (a medical doctor of 40 years' experience) an outspoken whistleblower of the AIDS hoax. In front of a gathering of about 30 alternative-medicine practitioners and several journalists, Willner stuck a needle in the finger of Andres, 27, a Fort Lauderdale student who says he has tested positive for HIV. Then, wincing, the 65-year-old doctor stuck himself. When asked why he would put his life on the line to make a point, Dr. Willner replied: "I do this to put a stop to the greatest murderous fraud in medical history. By injecting myself with HIV positive blood, I am proving a point. In this way it is my hope to expose the truth about HIV in the interest of all mankind." He tested negative for HIV multiple times.

2003: Hess and Unger failed to produce Varicella (chickenpox) in normal children by inoculating them upon the mucous membranes of the nose and throat with vesicle lymph and material collected from the nose and throat of patients with chickenpox or by inoculating them intracutaneously, subcutaneously, or intravenously with fresh vesicle lymph. Several observers (Lipschiltz, Meineri, and others) have made isolated attempts to inoculate human volunteers with Herpes Zoster (shingles), but always with negative results.

2012: In this experiment, people were sprayed with a cell culture directly up their noses. Two out of 15 people became ill. "Use of Human Influenza Challenge Model to Assess Person-to-Person Transmission: Proof-of-Concept Study." The Journal of Infectious Diseases, Killingley B, Enstone JE, Greatorex J, et al.

2020: In this experiment people were also sprayed with a cell culture directly up their noses. None of the 40 people became ill. "Minimal transmission in an Influenza A (H3N2) human challenge-transmission model within a controlled exposure environment. PLoS pathogens." Nguyen-Van-Tam JS, Killingley B, Enstone J, et al.

Bacteriologist Ilya Mechnicov (1845 − 1916), credited his health to eating tons of fermented yogurt bustling with bacteria. He experimented on himself, drinking Cholera. He didn't fall ill. Another participant did the same and didn't fall ill. Another participant fell severely ill, and he credited the disparity to the health of the participant's microbiome (terrain).

Prof Mac Von Pettenkoffer (1818 − 1901), along with his assistants, drank billions of Cholera during his classes, and nobody fell ill.

Dr. Thomas Powell injected himself with Cholera and "Bubonic Plague" germs and never fell ill.

Dr. Millicent Morden (1882-1955) wrote "Rabies Past/ Present". In her essay, Dr. Millicent references Dr. Woods' extensive experience with the Philadelphia dog pound. Dr. Woods, having dealt with over 150,000 rabid dogs over 25 years, observed that none of the pound workers who were bitten by the dogs ever developed rabies.[42]

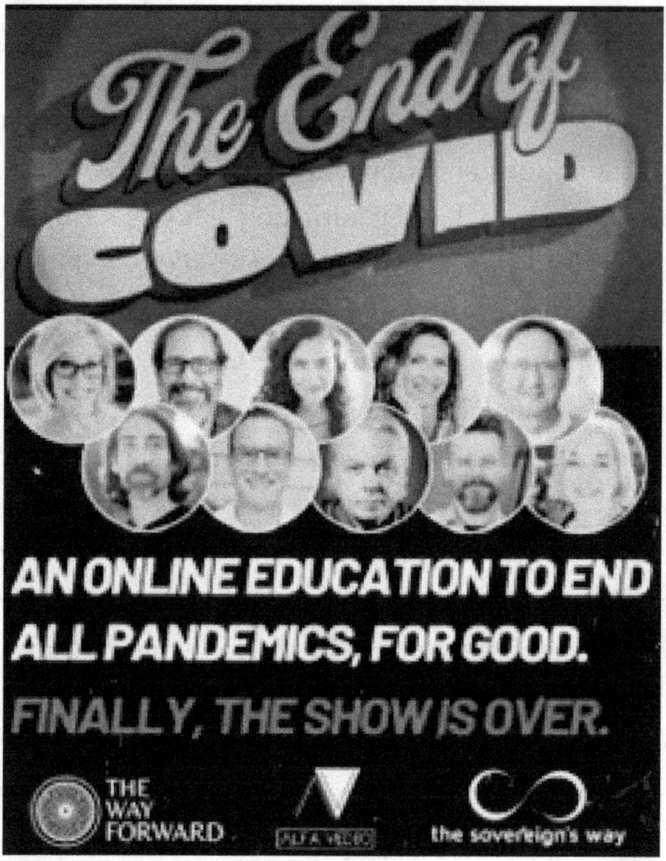
The End of
COVID
AN ONLINE EDUCATION TO END
ALL PANDEMICS, FOR GOOD.
FINALLY, THE SHOW IS OVER.
THE
WAY
FORWARD
the sovereign's way

CHAPTER 17

Where Does Contagion Come From?

❧

What is the expectation effect?

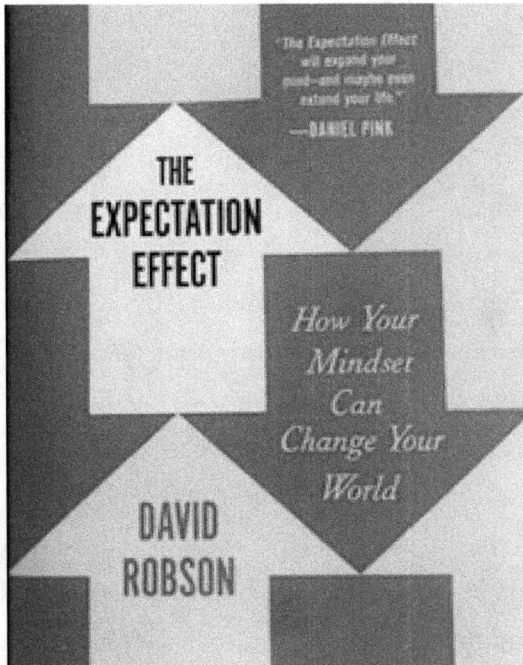

We've all heard about the placebo effect, where you think you're going to be better because of something, and so you are. But what about the nocebo effect? The term "nocebo" refers to a phenomenon where negative expectations or beliefs result in adverse effects or worsening of symptoms, even if the treatment or environment is harmless or inactive. In other words, it's the opposite of a placebo effect, where positive expectations lead to improvements. The Nocebo effect highlights the powerful influence of our mindset and beliefs on our physical and mental well-being.

There is an excellent book called "*The Expectation Effect*" that goes into the hundreds of studies that have been done to prove your beliefs and mindset can change your world. Not only your outer world but your inner world as well. We've all heard about the mind-body connection, right? Contagion is a perfect example of how people can get an expectation of catching something and manifest it to be true. This truth includes your health, both your symptoms and the disease itself. The expectation effect can even go so far as to create death in the body if the belief is strong enough. Consider the disease known as "Sudden Unexpected Nocturnal Death Syndrome."

"Starting in the late 1970s, the US Centers for Disease Control began to receive reports that a worrying number of recent Laotian immigrants were dying in their sleep. They were almost all male, aged between their mid-twenties and mid-forties, and most were from the persecuted Hmong ethnic group who had fled Laos after the rise to power of the Pathet Lao. For their loved ones, the only warning was the sound of them struggling for breath and, occasionally, a gasp, a moan, or a cry. By the time help arrived, however, they were already dead.

This became known as 'Sudden Unexpected Nocturnal Death Syndrome.' Autopsies could find no evidence of mental or dietary health issues. At its peak, the mortality rate was so high among these Hmong men that more lives were lost than all other top five causes of death combined. Investigations discovered that in their native land of Laos, the Hmong men could ask a shaman to make a protective necklace or sacrifice an animal to appease ancestors whose job it was to fend off evil demons roaming the world at night. The immigrants were without their rituals, and without the protection procured by the shaman, the men were vulnerable to attacks.

It was concluded that these men probably had sleep paralysis coupled with a panic so strong it could 'exacerbate a heart arrhythmia, leading to cardiac arrest.' The more Hmong that died, the more it created a contagious hysteria spreading throughout the people. The explanation is now accepted by many scientists."[43]

"In May of 2006, Portugal was beset by mysterious outbreaks of illness. The disease appeared to afflict only teenagers, who experienced dizziness, breathing difficulties, and skin rashes. Within a few days, around three hundred students across the country were affected. A virus or some kind of poisoning seemed the most likely pathogen, according to some experts; others believed it might be an allergic reaction to a certain kind of caterpillar or to dust in classrooms. None of the explanations seemed convincing, however. As one health expert remarked: 'I don't know any agent that is so selective it only attacks children.'

Inquiries eventually revealed that a popular teen soap, Morangos con Açucar (Strawberries with sugar), was to blame. In the days before the first reported case, the main characters on the show had been infected by a life-threatening virus that had led to very similar symptoms. Somehow, the 'virus' had jumped from the small screen to a handful of viewers, creating real physical symptoms, despite the fact that the illness in the program was totally fictional. Those children then passed it on to their classmates, leading to the cases multiplying. Portuguese adults were unlikely to have been dedicated viewers of the melodrama—and were less embedded in the teens' social networks—so they were less likely to develop the disease."[44]

"*The Expectation Effect*" is an awesome book filled with hundreds of similar studies that help to explain the contagion phenomenon. Your expectations can play a huge part in manifesting an illness or condition. Any time you see someone coughing, what goes through your mind? A cough is also very similar to a DOG BARKING! What goes through your mind when someone sneezes? Now you can think *happy thoughts and well wishes* to the person coughing and sneezing because they are in a healing phase!

The next time someone is sick around you, try to remember what you now know. You can't catch anything…unless…you think you can! Let go of the FEAR!

CHAPTER 18

German New Medicine, Another Explanation for Contagion and Disease

꙳

We'll unearth another explanation for contagion. Let us explain German New Medicine (GNM), The Five Biological Laws of Nature, and the story of how it was discovered.

The story goes like this. Dr. Ryke Hamer was the head internist at the cancer clinic at the University of Munich in Germany. He invented several medical devices that made him a great deal of money. Dr. Hamer and his wife (who was also a doctor) were planning on opening a free clinic for the poor in Italy. In 1978, they decided to take a trip with their four kids. When they were on their vacation, their oldest 16-year-old son, Dirk, was tragically shot by, of all people, the last monarch of Italy, Prince Victor Emmanuel of Savoy. Dirk lived for four months before he finally succumbed to his afflictions and died in his father's arms.

After agonizing over his son's death for several months afterward, Dr. Hamer was (to his surprise) diagnosed with testicular cancer. Shortly after, his wife was diagnosed with breast cancer as well! Even though they had both been very healthy. He started to wonder if their cancers had any relation to the tragedy of their son. So, Dr. Hamer went back to the cancer clinic at the University of Munich and started doing interviews and brain scans of all the cancer patients he attended. He started to see patterns. He found that every time someone got cancer, it followed an unexpected, shocking, and isolating event. There wasn't one case that did not follow a pattern. He also determined that each type of cancer developed after a very specific type of shocking event.

Then, one evening, as he was the attending physician in an Emergency Department, a patient was brought in unconscious and was assumed to be having a heart attack. The doctors rushed the gentleman off to have a CT scan (Computed Tomography) done on his brain. When Dr. Hamer viewed the CT scan, he noticed small concentric circles in the exact part of the brain that controls the heart rhythms. He realized the brain had a reaction in the corresponding organ relay, and those reactions linked to the diseased organ. These reactions can be seen in CT scans of the head!

He could look at a brain scan and see where in the brain the organ disease or cancer was being controlled. Not only that, but he could also tell with 100% accuracy what symptoms would occur and when the patient had gone into healing. He confirmed his discoveries with over 40,000 case studies. He developed the science of what is called German New Medicine and The Five Biological Laws of Nature.

He was so excited about his evidence and the fact that he had established not only a theory but actual laws that were later reproducible by other doctors! He went to his colleagues and tried to present his findings in a thesis. And guess what?? To his shock, they completely rejected even looking at his findings. They had the Semmelweis Reflex! This is an unprecedented case in the history of universities! Dr. Hamer was in for another shock. They gave him an ultimatum. He could discontinue his research or be fired from the cancer institute. He *stood his ground* and was dismissed. He went into private practice, where he continued his research. Hundreds of patients wrote to health officials to stand up for him and protest on his behalf. None of the letters were answered, and most were returned unopened.

In 1989, at age 54, they stripped him of his medical license on the grounds that he would not renounce his findings and would not prescribe chemotherapy to his cancer patients. In 1997, he was put in prison for giving three people medical advice. They put him in jail twice for over three years for practicing medicine without a license. While he was in jail, they confiscated 6500 patient records for condemning evidence. The prosecutor was forced to admit in his trial that of his 6500 terminally ill patients, 6000 were still alive after five years. He had over 90% success rate with terminally ill patients. The conventional approach of chemo, radiation, and surgery has a **less than 10% survival rate** with terminal cancers.

Why do you think the medical industry was so determined to silence Dr. Hamer? Was it the Semmelweis reflex, and they were just threatened by new ideas? Or was it a fear of losing control of the extremely profitable medical industry that uses drugs and surgery to make its profits?

Not everyone in medicine and academia has been afraid to validate Dr. Hamer's German New Medicine by looking at it. Here are some of the findings of verifiable documents and medical researchers.

Dr. Robert Guinée has been practicing GNM since the 1990s, and he is a direct protégé of Dr Ryke Hamer. Dr Guinée wrote a book in French based on Dr Hamer's work. As of this publication, the book is being translated into English and should be available soon.

The English title is *"Diseases, Memories of Evolution"* by Dr. Robert Guinée; based on the work of Doctor R.G. Hamer (French title: Maladies, mémoires de l'évolution / Dr Robert Guinée; basé sur les travaux du Docteur R.G. Hamer)[45]

Ilsedora Laker is also a direct protégé of Dr Ryke Hamer. Her blogs and seminars can be found on her website, www. gnmonlineseminars.com

The following is from Ilsedora Laker's blog "Treatment in the GNM":

"The discovery of the five biological laws is really more along the lines of a new natural science. For the first time in the history of medicine we can explain the origin of disease and understand that what we interpret as an illness or disease is not a mistake of nature. To find a 'cure' we don't have to try to find a way to manipulate this or that gene to 'correct' the problem or even find the miracle drug that will cure cancer once and for all.

The answer to dealing with all of our so-called illnesses is within ourselves and understanding what event in our life's experience gave us the physical response.

Sure, we can use remedies to make ourselves more comfortable and to try to alleviate symptoms, but they are *not the cure*.

60% of all of our so-called illnesses only occur when the conflict shock is *solved*.

The amazing thing about this particular approach is that when we are dealing with chronic conditions, which are mostly really prolonged healing phases (60% of all of our so-called illnesses only occur when the conflict shock is solved), the moment we find the conflict shock a physical shift takes place and, in many cases, an immediate alleviation of symptoms!

In other cases, if the physical problem is caused by conflict activity, for example, a functional problem like MS or a blood sugar problem, it must pass through the healing phase before healing is completed.

Our approach to the treatment in GNM is not random.

…Every health concern (outside of poisoning) known to man is caused by a specific kind of biological conflict, so the GNM consultant already knows what kind of unanticipated event to look for. This is the treatment in the GNM."[46]

These documents can be found on www.learninggnm.com

1984: A doctor from the (Cardiology Clinic, Vienna), and two radiologists, both from the University of Vienna, Austria, tested eight patients based on Dr. Hamer's findings regarding the correlation between a heart attack, a territorial loss conflict, and alterations in the brain in form of a so-called Hamer Focus (HH).

The committee members acknowledged through their signatures that, in accordance with the (First Biological Law) all heart attacks had occurred after the territorial conflict was resolved.

1988: Univ. Prof. Dr. Birkmeyer and Dr. Rozkydal (both Vienna, Austria) tested the First Biological Law on seven patients, supervised by five physicians. The result: 100 % accuracy.

1989: At a medical conference in Munich (Germany), 17 doctors tested the Five Biological Laws on 27 patients. The results: 100% accuracy.

1990: 6 patients were tested in Namur (Belgium) supervised by 17 medical doctors. The result: 100% accuracy.

1990: During an international medical conference in Burgau (Austria) 20 patients were tested, supervised by 30 doctors. The result: 100% accuracy.

1992: Dr. Stemmann, doctor of pediatrics and member of the **Medical Faculty of the University of Düsseldorf**, Germany, tested at a medical conference in Germany on May 23-24, 1992 the reproducibility of Dr. Hamer's discoveries based on 24 cases. On average, each case presented four to five diseases, including cancers, brain tumors, leukemia, multiple sclerosis, epilepsy, sarcoma, diabetes, infections, tuberculosis, and mental illnesses. The committee found the Five Biological Laws of the "New Medicine" to be 100% accurate in all 24 cases.

1993: Dr. Stangl, president of the Medical Officer Association of Lower Austria, tested the Five Biological Laws on 250 cases. The result: 100% agreement with Dr. Hamer's findings.

1998: The **Medical Faculty of the University of Slovakia** tested seven patients with 20 specific medical conditions at the Sainte Elisabeth Institute of Oncology at Bratislava and the Oncology unit of the Hospital of Slovakia. As stated in the official certification: "The objective was to establish whether Dr. Hamer's system of medicine could be verified by using a scientific method to show that his results are repeatable." This has been the case 100% of the time.

On July 12, **2011**, the **Government of Nicaragua** officially recognized German New Medicine® as a medical therapy.[47]

CHAPTER 19

How Does German New Medicine Work?

❦

Each of the 5 Biological laws of German New Medicine outlines an important principle in the causation of disease, its different phases, the place in the brain where it affects us (which can easily be identified on a brain scan), the specific organ or tissue in the body that will be affected, and finally how the process of healing occurs with an unbelievable natural repair and cleanup process! We call them Biological Laws of Nature because Dr. Hamer showed us that they are not from one angle of interpretation. They are not only psychological, only the brain or only the body. They are a composite of all of these.

Biological Law #1: Every disease originates from a serious life trauma or shock that is unexpected, sudden, intense, and isolating. Dr Hamer coined the term Dirk Hamer Syndrome (DHS) to put a name to this kind of conflict *in honor of his son*

Dirk. This conflict shock affects ***simultaneously*** three levels of **our system:**

1. The psyche
2. The brain
3. The corresponding tissue in the body.

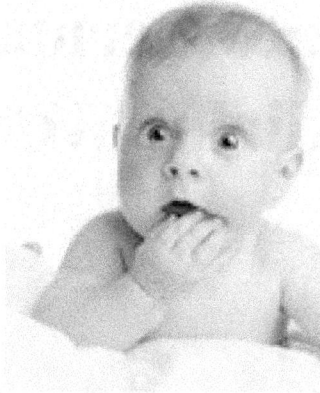

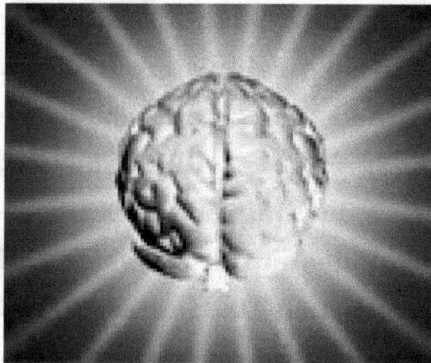

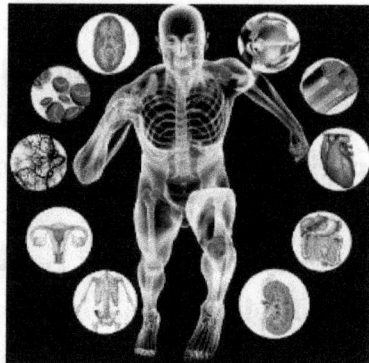

+

+

For example, let's start with nature. If a deer is chased by a predator, it will feel the sudden conflict shock of "my life is in danger," and the brain stem of the deer will instantly send a message to the lung tissue to grow more lung cells so that the deer can take in more oxygen and thus is more likely to get away and survive.

In the case of a human that experiences a life-threatening shock, such as a cancer diagnosis, or as in the case of millions of people feeling threatened during WW2, the result will be the same. The brain stem that controls the lung will send a message to the lungs to produce more lung tissue to deal with the shock. In conventional medicine, more lung tissue or growths are diagnosed as lung cancer. What is the first thing we do when we get a frightening surprise? WE GASP FOR AIR! But there's more to the story...

At the Psyche level: Let's say your doctor gives you the news that you have a brain tumor. You suffer a death fright conflict. This sudden and unexpected life trauma creates a feeling of isolation and a fight-or-flight response. For disease to occur, the state of distress must remain *unresolved* long enough for the corresponding reaction on the physical level to be detected either as a symptom or by medical tests.

Our typical worries, when known and expected, even if just for a few instants before the shock occurs, do not cause a lesion in the brain that can then lead to disease. But if we tend to worry, it can certainly predispose us to overreacting and triggering a survival response.

Brain: A lesion appears in the brain at a location related to the specific nature of each shock. It is seen on a brain scan as a bullseye. Imagine seeing a pebble dropped in a pond. What do we typically see? Concentric circles in the water. That is exactly what happens in our brain when we perceive a shock! Our brain is programmed to initiate survival programs depending on which center is affected. These *survival programs* evolved as we as a species evolved. In the case of a death fright, it occurs in the brain stem.

In the case of a separation conflict, it occurs in the cortex of the brain (the ectoderm germ layer). Dr. Hamer had testicular cancer, which occurs in the cerebral medulla.

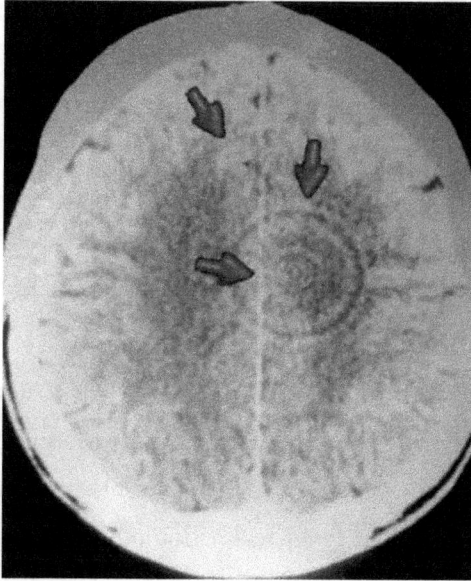

Dr. R G Hamer Library

Body: At the instant of the shock, the cells at the location of the brain lesion receive the signal of distress and transmit it to the respective body tissue that is in charge of assisting in such situations. A biological response is triggered – one that can help us to either resolve the crisis or which can buy us some time in order to find a solution. This survival mechanism involves an increase or decrease of cells in the involved tissue or a change in regular functions. We refer to it as an adaption or "tissue response."

In the case of Dr. Hamer, he suffered a "profound loss of a loved one conflict." The cerebrum immediately got the message and sent the alert to the testicles. The testicles went through cell loss for the purpose of replenishment during the healing stage.

Biologically, the new cells in the testicles actually form a cyst, which will produce even more testosterone than previously to attract a female, make up for the loss of a child or mate, and produce new offspring. Did you get that? The new cyst that forms actually produces testosterone in order to help create more offspring. So you see, nature isn't out to get us. It is ALWAYS there to support us!

We'll cover all of the **Biological Laws of Nature Dr Hamer discovered** *in the last chapter.*

Now that you have been introduced to GNM, let's talk about contagions like colds and flu.

CHAPTER 20

Colds and Flus Explained

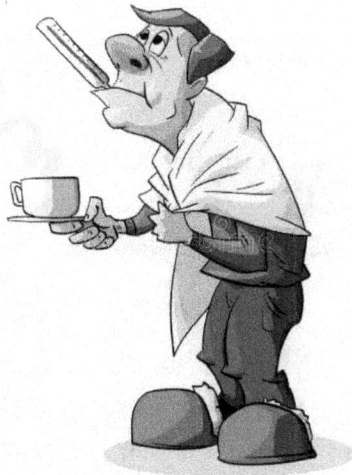

❧

Dr. Ryke Hamer, the founder of German New Medicine (GNM), has found in his research that some colds begin as what he would call a "stink conflict." When there is something that figuratively "stinks," your brain sends an instant message to the nose to clear out tissue to deal with the stink (smell less of the stink). When the conflict is resolved, your body will replace the tissue. In other words, when you feel less stress or when your life doesn't "stink" as much, you will start having healing symptoms. You will have a stuffy nose with inflammation. Your nose will run, and you may have a headache and a fever because the area is healing a "stink conflict." Think of the last time you had a runny nose. What stress did you go through before that? What was something that made you mad (incensed?) or that you subconsciously labeled "this stinks"? Or, possibly, you were confronted with a disgusting odor! Think of how our forefathers got around in the streets of towns! On horseback! Have you ever been too close to someone speaking to you who had poor dental hygiene?

Other explanations for Flus and colds are the way your body releases toxic build-up or resolves a period of mental or emotional stress. Usually, we have more toxins of stress, chemicals, food, and alcohol during the holidays or "flu season," so it's common for people to "catch a cold or the flu" at that time. We are not catching anything from someone else…We are *reacting psychologically and biologically in the same way as those close to us are.* We actually can "catch" the same stress or toxins as other people, and we feel FEAR! Colds and flu are also a lot more common at the time when trees have released their leaves. When the trees lose their leaves, they are not taking toxins out of the air or giving as much oxygen. This can lead to our own toxic build-up, which is why we often get colds or flu in the first place. We need to detox.

Dr. Ryke Hamer MD states, "Contrary to the common belief, (colds and flu) are not at all related to viruses but rather to an *"indigestible morsel conflict"* and *"territorial anger conflict"* experienced simultaneously by a group of people (city residents, villagers, family members, colleagues, schoolmates, roommates, friends) who share the same anger-environment (at home, at work, in daycare, in kindergarten, at school, in nursing homes, etc.).” At first, the word “morsel” probably sounds odd, but it really is the right word to use because it can refer to any small piece or thing.

Think about it: children are sent off to their first daycare experience. Many come down with a “cold” or sickness several days or weeks after they start. Many experience a new conflict (*fear* being one) and get triggered by the new environment that is not their familiar home, the separation from their parents, and meeting strange new faces. Once they *get over their conflict,* they cough, sneeze, and blow their noses because their bodies are breaking down the small cell over-growths. We attribute this to “catching germs,” and something must be “going around.” The children are, in reality, just experiencing the same stress. This stress creates an environment in the body that would be labeled a dis-ease. As soon as the child feels safer and no longer feels any fear, the dis-ease build-up is released, giving them cold or flu symptoms.

Large psychological stressors in the environment, such as fear of war or deadly “viruses,” can trigger regional dis-ease followed by a “stomach flu” outbreak in the affected population after the conflict has been resolved. Stomach Flu epidemics typically occur after natural disasters, such as floods or earthquakes, during the resolution phase.”[48]

We are trained our whole life to stay away from sick people so we don’t get sick. Or we need to stay home when we’re sick so we don’t pass anything along. But real scientific studies do not support this, as we have shown earlier. Much of what we do is based on propaganda started by Louis Pasteur and the un-reproducible Germ Theory. This is to perpetuate the selling of drugs and vaccines. And who funds the propaganda? Those who make money on drugs and vaccine sales. Follow the money, my friend!

Think of the lepers in bible times and in stories of Mother Teresa's nuns. Did any of the disciples or nuns ever contract leprosy?

A study was done in February of 1921 by the *Hygienic Laboratory #123* of the US government. (Another disgustingly brave experiment). The study was done where they tried to contaminate 62 Navy personnel with the flu in every possible way. They took sputum from influenza cases and sprayed it down their throats and on their food. They kept the Navy personnel in constant contact with flu patients. The conclusion of the study showed "no appreciable reactions" in any of the 62 subjects. *Nothing* showed that the subjects of the experiment caught anything from anyone![49]

We are trained to believe that a cold "virus" is transmitted through your spit or mucus particles when you cough, sneeze, or just breathe. The particles are thought to be inhaled by another person, who then becomes infected by the virus, which travels through their body to the affected part of the lung tissue. The transmission of viral particles has never, ever been observed or proven!

Remember, germs and viruses are not the bad guys! They are always at the scene of the fire, but they are not the arsonists.

A very thorough analysis of all diseases can be found in Dr. Hamer's work.

We strongly encourage you to visit the following websites:

www.gnmonlineseminars.com and www.learninggnm.com for an in-depth look at German New Medicine (GNM) and any diagnosis you are curious about, from cancers to canker sores!

Dr. Ryke Hamer, MD, proves in his work called The Five Biological Laws that germs don't cause disease but instead *play a vital role during the healing phase.* Dr. Hamer, MD concluded about germs after 30 years of research, "*They live in harmony with all organisms of the ecological milieu in which they have developed over millions of years.*"[50]

CHAPTER 21

Has a Measles Virus ever been isolated?

❧

Dr. Stefan Lanka offered $100,000 to anyone in Germany who produced genuine scientific proof of the *measles virus*. In 2016, the courts in Germany found *no one had provided any of the necessary proof of a measles virus*. Seriously? We all know there's a measles virus, right? Wrong! It's never been isolated and injected in a healthy person and caused measles...EVER! There's a skin condition called measles. But it's NOT caused by a virus. It's a skin condition that derives from separation stress (conflict) and runs its course through a conflict phase and a healing phase (repair phase), as discovered by Dr. Ryke Gerd Hamer, the father of German New Medicine. The red bumps we see are visible symptoms of the body healing its own skin. Just a heads up! If you search the internet about Dr Lanka's court case, you will find many articles saying that he lost his case in court. However, after his team realized the judge hadn't read through all the evidence, Lanka appealed and WON![51]

The original term "smallpox" was a label given to anyone in previous centuries who presented with ANY form of a rash on the skin. Today, smallpox is labeled measles, chickenpox, or monkeypox.

"What we today call Chickenpox, Monkeypox, Scarlet Fever, Measles, Rubella, Herpes Zoster (shingles), Erythema Multiforme, Molluscum Contagiosum, Impetigo, Dermatitis, and so on were labels that were created to separate the previously unified term "Smallpox" for conditions accompanied by a rash." - Ekaterina Sugak, Naturopath www.ekaterinasugak.com[52]

CHAPTER 22

The Story of Masha and Dasha

❧

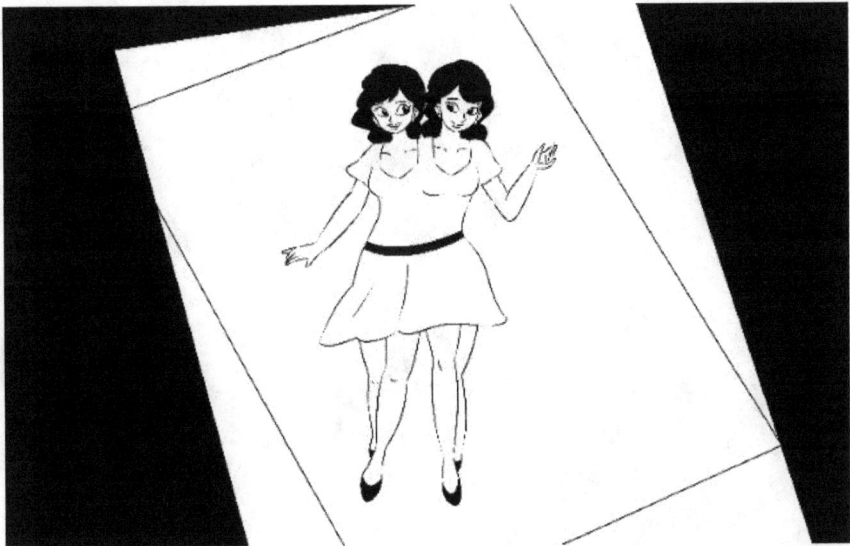

Picture this sad story about conjoined twins Masha and Dasha. Their new mother was told that they had died at birth. However, the truth was that they were sent to be studied at an institute near Moscow.

Because they shared the same blood, they should've experienced all the childhood diseases like measles, flu, and colds at the same time one of the two got sick. However, it was seen repeatedly that these diseases were experienced by each one of them at *different times*. Why is this so? Why did one become ill with a childhood disease, like measles, for example, while the other did not? The measles "bug" was assumed to be in both of their bodies, in their collective bloodstream. So why didn't they both get measles? Because measles is NOT *caused* by a virus or germ, and neither is the flu or cold! Review Chapter 20!

CHAPTER 23

What About Man-made "Viruses"?

❦

The word "virus" means poison. Most scientists think that viruses are attacking us to harm us as a poison due to the strong belief in the Germ Theory that has been propagated in every school. Scientists and chemists can make man-made poisons to harm and kill. But poisons and viruses aren't the same thing. Poisons are pollutants and biochemicals that are still not transferable by breathing or touching. Yes, they can inject them or even circulate them in the atmosphere, but don't be confused that they are made by your body or contagious! They are simply chemicals or manipulated genetic strands that act like poison. They are not naturally occurring "viruses." Remember, viruses are not alive; they don't fly around, they don't live on surfaces, and they don't attack you.

Once again, if your body has any toxins present, both bacteria and viruses and often fungus may be present to *clean up* the mess and remove or repair the damaged cells. Just as we wouldn't blame firemen for setting a fire at a burning house, we should not blame bacteria, viruses, or fungi for diseases. They are only trying to clean up the toxins by feeding on them to eliminate them from the diseased site or to repair and rebuild tissue that has been damaged. Think of them as *microsurgeons*.

CHAPTER 24

Has *Any Virus* Been Isolated?

❧

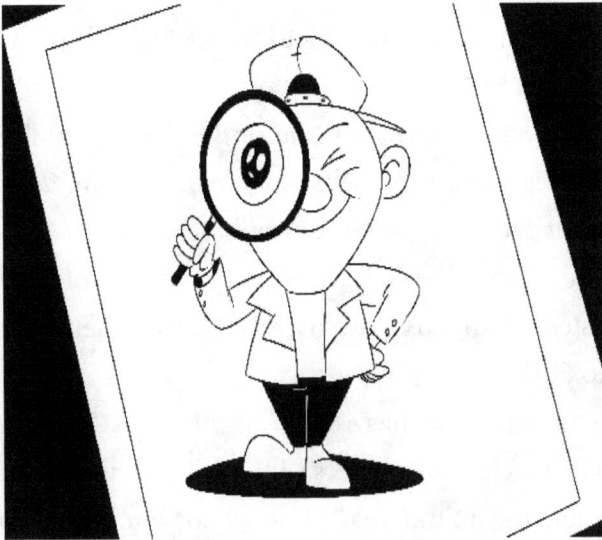

Viruses are so tiny that they can only be seen by an electron microscope and the atomic force microscope (1989). Although viruses were being blamed for diseases in the late 1800s, the electron microscope was not invented until 1931.

If scientists take a snapshot of any diseased tissue and look at it under an electron microscope, they will see bits of viruses because they are like sponges, which are there for cleanup. Scientists are witnessing dead cells with virus particles within them mixed with other dead cells (isolates) with viruses in them. They call this a virus "isolate" to make it sound as if they have something "isolated." But they don't!

Viruses are three times smaller than infrared rays. Their actual size is about 400 nm. This makes them ten times smaller than a Bacterium!

Their small size makes them the perfect suspect and scapegoat for any health crime. No one could actually see them or isolate them because even an electron microscope causes what's called nano-particulates. Scientists are looking at dead cellular debris that is bigger than viruses and too difficult to distinguish with certainty, let alone isolate to test.

Doctors never see viruses because they're too small to test, so instead, they test for antibodies, which can be seen. *There has never been a correlation between a specific virus and a specific antibody.* Antibodies will *always* be present if you have toxins in an area of the body that is being tested. It means absolutely nothing other than that the body has toxins!

To this day, no one has isolated a virus. A "virus isolate" is a term used in scientific papers. The titles of the reports sound convincing on the initial read, but when you read through the content of the report, they refer to Virus Like Particles (VLP)! That is not a virus! That is a combination of particles. That does not make it a virus.

And if you read further, you will note that, in many reports, this "isolate" has so much cellular debris added to it under a microscope it doesn't make sense! The isolate we see in the pictures includes dead tissue cells of sick animals and a handful of other viruses. A "virus isolate" is NOT an "isolated virus." This is important because *to <u>prove</u> a disease, you must have an isolated virus,* back to Koch's postulates.

What this means is that **no virus has ever been isolated!** The Measles virus, Polio virus, Diphtheria virus, Tetanus virus, Herpes virus, and HIV virus; none of these have EVER been isolated.

1954 marks the year when a scientist named John Enders essentially came up with protocols, which, when followed, would make it *appear* as if they had an "isolated virus" for any disease. Scientists can make it *appear* as if there is a new virus for any presentation within their lab.

Dr. Stefan Lanka said, **"In the course of my studies, I and others have not been able to find proof of the existence of disease-causing viruses anywhere."** Remember, Dr. Stefan Lanka offered $100,000 to anyone who could prove that the measles virus was isolated.[53]

Why is this important? Just to remind you, if you *can't* isolate the virus, you can't ever **prove** it causes disease. Plus, if you do any research, you will find that all the diseases blamed on viruses have often been diagnosed *with no* virus being present, and no control experiments are ever presented!

> **"Facts do not cease to exist because they are ignored."**
> **- Aldous Huxley**

In the awesome book *"VIRUS MANIA: How the Medical Industry Continually Invents Epidemics, Making Billion-Dollar Profits At Our Expense"* by Torsten Engelbrecht, Dr. Claus Kohnlein, Dr. Samantha Bailey, MD, Dr. Stefano Scoglio, MD,[24] there are over 2000 research articles saying the same thing. The book is full of facts regarding the bogus virus theory of disease.[54]

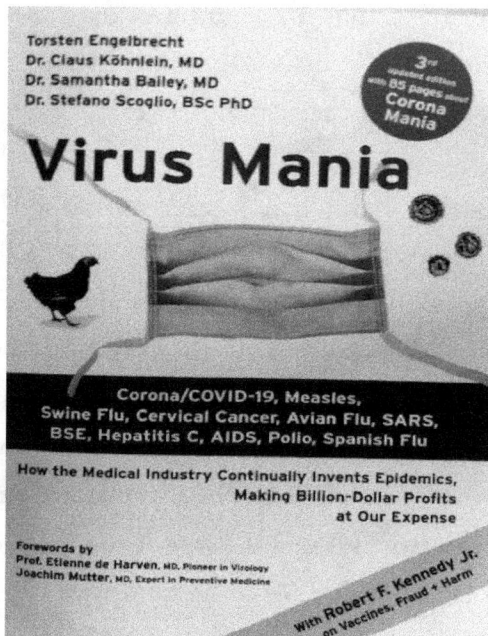

Most research is paid for by those who make money on the outcome. The French government supported Louis Pasteur's research and paid him to promote germ theory and then vaccinations because they were making a huge profit. And now we know his work was fraudulent!

If you look at today's research, it is paid for by Big Pharma in one way or another. There is rarely independent research, and the conclusions are bought and paid for.

Today, most books on health are still written with the idea that bacteria and viruses cause disease. Unfortunately, it's misinformation that has been repeated for 150 years. Anytime you hear about a virus or a bacteria, try to think of what toxin (physical, mental, social, or spiritual) actually caused that disease process. Anytime you hear about an infection, think of what *toxin* caused the bacteria, virus, or fungus to show up.

"It should be clear from this discussion that no disease is caused by a virus" - Dawn Lester and David Park, "*What Really Makes You Ill?*" [55]

"The health authorities are no longer maintaining that any virus whatsoever purportedly causing disease has been *directly proven* to exist." Dr. Robert Mendelsohn MD[56]

"Life is an incredibly complex interdependence of matter and energy among millions of species beyond and within our own skin." - Dr. Margulis [57]

"This germ theory of the Dark Age is nothing but a deliberate *mass insanity* pushed upon society to gain profit and power. By acting against microbes as a medical establishment dictate, one is actually helping to dig one's own grave, while paying someone else to show where to dig. This insanity must end." - Dr. William Trebing [58]

We were all led to believe in school that these "bad germs" are single-minded opportunists who work for your persistent demise. Nothing could be further from the truth. They are part of the body's defense mechanism to clean house, purify the system, and return us to homeostasis (balance).

CHAPTER 25

What About the Polio Virus?

❧

Scientists tried to prove that polio is contagious by doing extensive studies on monkeys. All of the studies were failures until they finally resorted to <u>drilling a hole</u> in a monkey's skull and injecting a ground-up piece of spinal cord from a sick child with polio into the monkey's brain. When the monkey became paralyzed, they reported that they succeeded in showing polio was contagious! Drilling a hole in someone's head would paralyze anyone! This study did not prove anything, yet it is used as one of the main studies trying to prove Polio contagion.

Another cornerstone study for the polio "virus" theory was started in 1908 by scientists Karl Landsteiner and Erwin Popper. The WHO claimed their experiments were a milestone in the obliteration of polio. Listen to the account of the ridiculous experiments used to validate the use of polio vaccines!

Landsteiner and Popper took a diseased piece of spinal marrow from a lame nine-year-old boy. They chopped it up, dissolved it in water, and injected one or two whole cups of it into the *abdominal cavities* of two test monkeys: one died, and the other became permanently paralyzed. Their studies were plagued by a mind-boggling range of basic problems. First, the "glop" they poured into the animals was not even infectious since the paralysis didn't appear in the monkeys and guinea pigs given the alleged "virus soup" to *drink* or in those that had it *injected* into their extremities. [59]

Shortly after, researchers Simon Flexner and Paul Lewis experimented with a comparable mixture, **injecting this into monkeys' brains.[60] Next, they brewed a new soup from the brains of these monkeys and put the mix into another monkey's head. This monkey indeed became ill!**

But this experiment shows no proof of a viral infection! The glop used cannot be termed an isolated virus, even with all the will in the world!! Nobody could have seen any virus, as the electron microscope wasn't invented until 1931! Also, Flexner and Lewis did not disclose the ingredients of their "injection soup." By 1948, it was still unknown "how the polio virus invades humans," as expert John Paul of Yale University stated at an international poliomyelitis congress in New York City.[61]

Believe it or not, this is the ONE experiment that is held up as *proving* that polio is caused by a virus that invades humans! They injected the goop soup into a monkey's brain to cause paralysis and thus link polio to a virus!

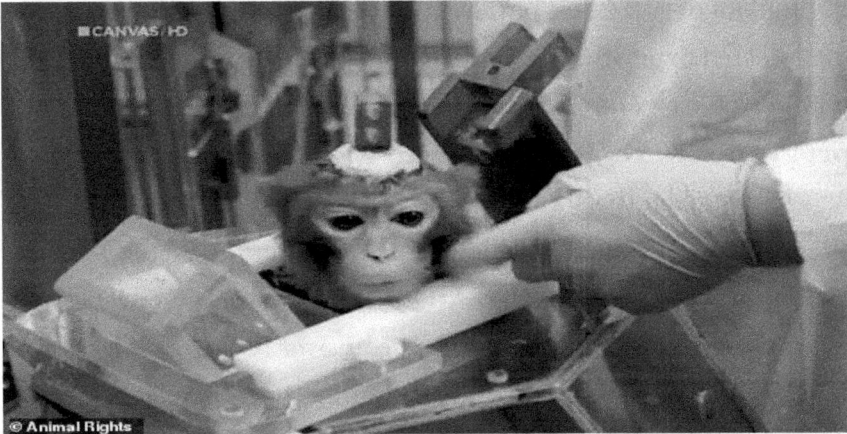

However, not all scientists were impressed.

In 1941, expert scientists reported in the scientific journal ARCHIVES of Pediatrics that "Human poliomyelitis **has not** been shown conclusively to be a *contagious disease*."[62] Well, if any scientist read the previous experiment, they should have ALL concluded that!

Despite this fact, a Polio vaccine was developed. In 1955, Salk's Vaccine was celebrated nationwide as a substance that protected against polio outbreaks. However, one year earlier, in 1954, Bernice Eddy, who oversaw the US government's vaccine safety tests, reported that the Salk vaccine *had caused severe paralyzes in test monkeys*. How does the US government solve these findings? Bernice Eddy was shortly after forced to *give up* her position and polio research.

Within only two weeks, the number of polio cases among vaccinated children had climbed to nearly 200. In May 1955, Carl Eklund, the US government's highest authority on viruses, said, "only vaccinated children had been afflicted by polio. And only in areas where no polio cases had been reported for close to a year! In nine out of ten cases, paralysis for the polio vaccine appeared in the injected arm. In New York, Rhode Island, and Wisconsin, the number of cases of paralysis **jumped to 500% after vaccine programs were administered**. Most frequently in the arm which was given the shot!" [63]

Guess what Polio, Aseptic Meningitis, the Flu, Lyme Disease, Whooping cough, Lupus, and AIDS (Acquired Immune Deficiency Syndrome) all have in common? The answer is: *THEY ALL HAVE IDENTICAL SYMPTOMS*!! The only difference between them is that their symptoms are *switched around* a bit in the order of what symptom is listed first when referenced in any popular diagnostic text. Essentially, all these diseases are part of the same process, which renders them practically identical.

CHAPTER 26

So, What Did Cause Polio?

The truth about Polio is twofold. In the late 1940s and early 1950s, the government sprayed yards, orchards, and parks with a DDT pesticide (glyphosates) to kill moths. This was a *lead-arsenate* toxic concoction that is known to cause nerve and muscle damage exactly like the "Polio" symptoms. Lucky for us, they stopped spraying yards with this toxic chemical in 1955. Lucky *and profitable* for Big Pharma, they came up with a Polio vaccine right at the end of the time they stopped spraying (1955) so they could claim that the Polio vaccine was a success.

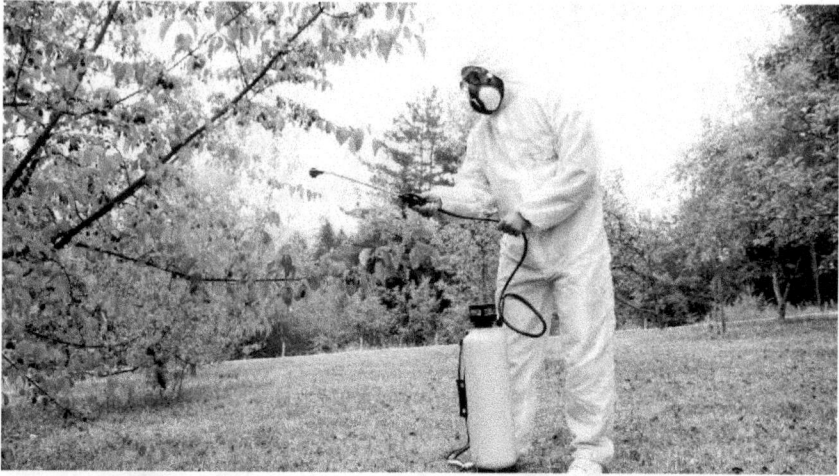

The other thing they cleverly did was force doctors to change their diagnostic tactics. Any child after 1959 with polio-like symptoms was to be diagnosed with Acute Flaccid Paralysis (AFP). "Doctors are instructed not to look for the Polio virus itself, as 'the virus is very hard to find.' Instead, this task is to be left to WHO and the other governmental agencies that inspect turds (doctors are to send in two). This would've been comical if it were not so tragically deceptive," says Janine Roberts in *"Fear of the Invisible: A Hidden Epidemic."* [64]

She continues, "Under these new rules, patients previously diagnosed with paralytic polio were re-diagnosed. When patients in Detroit, diagnosed as having paralytic Polio during 1958 epidemic, were re-tested as required by the new rule, 49% were found not to have the Polio virus and were therefore told they did not have Polio. I did not know how to characterize this except as an incredible act of medical fraud."[65] So much for Polio vaccines eradicating Polio. They only eradicated the diagnosis and continued the shell game!

"Health officials convinced the Chinese to rename the bulk of their polio to Guillain-Barré Syndrome (GBS). A study found that the new disorder (Chinese Paralytic syndrome) and GBS was really Polio. After mass vaccination in 1971, reports of Polio went down but GBS increased about 10-fold! In the WHO Polio vaccine eradication in the Americas, there were 930 cases of paralytic disease all called Polio. Five years later, at the end of the campaign, *roughly 2000 cases of paralytic disease occurred but only 6 of them were called Polio.* The rate of paralytic disease doubled, but the disease definition changed so drastically that hardly any of it was called Polio anymore." [66]

Unfortunately, government agencies and corporations continue to spray different nerve poisons all over the world as herbicides and pesticides and cause neurological problems in children.[67]

The inventor of the Polio vaccine Jonas Salk is quoted as saying that over two-thirds of the Polio cases after 1976 were caused by his Salk vaccine![68]

CHAPTER 27

What About the Spanish Flu of 1918 That Killed 20-50 Million People?

❧

We have all heard that the Spanish Flu killed 20,000,000 to 50,000,000 people. It was considered one of the deadliest pandemics of all time. But was it actually contagious or a "flu"?

One medical team in Boston, working for the United States public health service, tried to infect 100 healthy volunteer sailors between the ages of 18 and 25. Their efforts were impressive and made entertaining reading:

"We collected the material and mucous secretions from the mouth, nose, and throats of sick people and transferred this to our volunteers. We always obtained this material in the same way. The patient, with fever, in bed, had a large shallow tray-like arrangement before him or her, and we washed out one nostril with some sterile salt solutions, using perhaps 5cc, which is allowed to run into the tray, and that nostril is blown vigorously into the tray. This is repeated with the other nostril. The patient then gargles with some of the solution. Next, we obtained some bronchial mucus through the coughing, and then we swapped the mucus surface of each naris and also the mucus surface of the throat... Each one of the volunteers... received 6cc of the mixed stuff that I have described. They received it into each nostril; received it in the throat and on the eye; and when you think that 6cc is all that was used, you will understand that some of it was swallowed. None of them became ill."

In a further experiment with new volunteers and donors, the salt solution was eliminated, and with cotton swabs, the material was transferred directly from nose to nose and from throat to throat, using donors on the first, second, or third day of the disease.

"None of these volunteers who received the material thus directly transferred from cases took sick in any way...all of the volunteers received at least two, and some of them three 'shots' as they expressed it.

Then, we collected a lot of mucus material from the upper respiratory tract and filtered it through Mandler filters. This filtrate was injected into ten volunteers, each one receiving 3.5cc subcutaneously, and none of these took sick in any way."

Then, a further attempt was made to transfer the disease "in the natural way," using fresh volunteers and donors:

"The volunteer was led up to the bedside of the patient; he was introduced. He sat down beside the bed of the patient. They shook hands, and by instructions, he got as close as he conveniently could, and they talked for five minutes. At the end of five minutes, the patient breathed out as hard as he could, while the volunteer, muzzle to muzzle (in accordance with his instructions about two inches between the two), received this expired breath, and at the same time was breathing in as the patient breathed out... after they had done this five times, the patient coughed directly into the face of the volunteer, face to face, five different times... [Then] he moved to the next patient whom we had selected, and repeated this, and so on, until this volunteered had had that sort of contact with ten different cases of Influenza in different stages of the disease, mostly fresh cases, none of them more than three days old... **none of them took sick in any way**."

NOT ONE SAILOR CAME DOWN WITH THE SPANISH FLU!" - *"Invisible Rainbow"* by Arthur Firstenberg [69]

How do you explain that?

The Spanish Flu was NOT contagious. Yes, many people died, but it was not caused by a contagious virus (because viruses or bacteria are NOT contagious, nor do they cause disease)! There were so many culprits other than a virus. The most likely being the extreme stress caused by the announcement of WWI combined with a bacterial meningitis vaccine containing mercury, aluminum, and other toxins. This vaccine was given to millions both in our country and around the world.

The radio wave was first released around the world in 1917 with the invention of new radar equipment. The symptoms that people were experiencing during the Spanish Flu included hemorrhaging blood from all different parts of the body. These symptoms are consistent with what is known about the effects of radio waves on blood.

There were also extreme sanitation problems and little nutrition due to the abysmal food supply following the war. These conditions also led to millions of deaths preceded by flu-like symptoms.

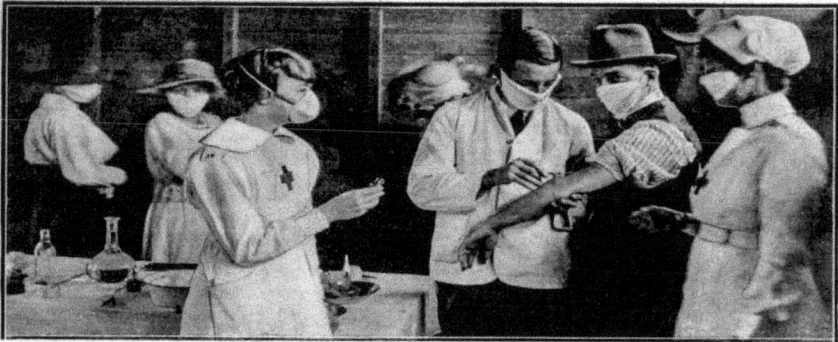

And guess what? The Spanish Flu did not start in Spain! They were the only country uncensored during WWI, so they were the only country reporting deaths, and thus, they were blamed for causing it. And the reason the Spanish Flu has never been corrected is that the name helps disguise the origin of the pandemic, which was actually the US.

This next revelation could be a shock to hear...

The main origin of the pandemic may have involved a **vaccine experiment** on US Soldiers; the US much prefers to label it The Spanish Flu instead of The Fort Riley Vaccine of 1918, or something similar. The Spanish Flu possibly started at Fort Riley, Kansas, where this experimental vaccine was given by the Rockefeller Institute. The Rockefeller Institute was established back in 1901.

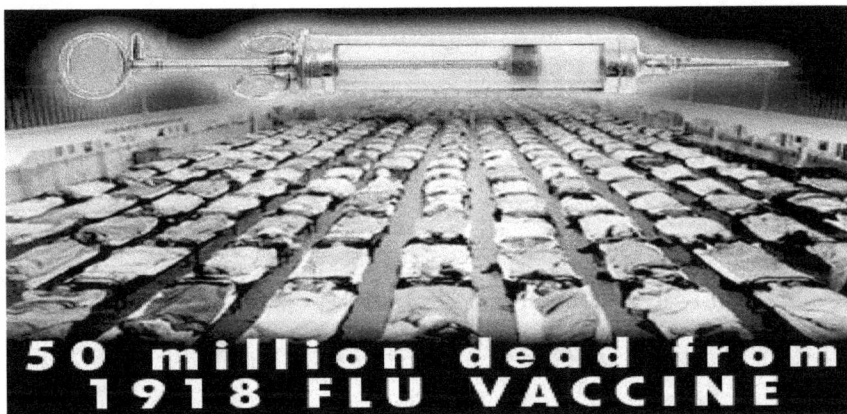

50 million dead from
1918 FLU VACCINE

"The American Rockefeller Institute for Medical Research and its experimental bacterial meningococcal vaccine may have killed 50,000,000-100,000,000 people in 1918-1919" is a far less effective sales slogan than the overly simplistic 'vaccines save lives.'" – Kevin Barry, the President of First Freedoms, Inc. a 501.c.3. He is a former federal attorney, a representative at the United Nations Headquarters in New York, and the author of "Vaccine Whistleblower: Exposing Autism Research Fraud at the CDC."[70]

Remember that bacteria and viruses will appear whenever toxins are present? If you were unfortunate enough to be a soldier or part of the military staff in 1918, you would have been injected with the experimental bacterial meningitis vaccine. The experimental vaccine, derived from horses, comprised toxins like mercury and aluminum, along with horse serum. When you're injected with toxins, you're bound to feel sick. Combining the heavy metals in the vaccines with the newly released worldwide radio wave of electricity was deadly.

And that was reported again and again. Nausea, diarrhea, vomiting, and often death... makes sense, right? So, did the vaccinations stop? No, of course not. The Rockefeller Institute for Health kindly sent vaccinations overseas to "help" the rest of the world. It was big money.

There were far more deaths from the Spanish Flu than from any actual war. If there was any desire to reduce the world population and make money, vaccines were successful. The Rockefeller Institute of Health discovered vaccines were better for business than war. They could *appear as if they were helping people* yet be killing them.

Another major culprit was the HUGE amount of fear and emotional trauma that can affect large numbers of people simultaneously and make them sick.

Have you noticed there has never been another Spanish Flu viral epidemic? Because it was a made-up flu virus! You will have to look for the references in the back to research this on your own. Google has removed a lot of information about the Spanish flu after the coronavirus was *announced*.

If you have gotten vaccines in your life, we are happy if you have not had any complications. However, there is a multitude of evidence that vaccines have caused many deaths.

CHAPTER 28

What About the HIV and AIDS Epidemic?

❦

Guess what? There are over 1500 peer-reviewed articles disputing the claim that HIV is linked to AIDS (Acquired Immune Deficiency Syndrome) or that HIV existed at all! Look at www.virusmyth.org and www.virusmyth.com for more research. According to the book "*Virus Mania*," there are many researchers, including the "discoverers" of the HIV (theory), Luc Montagnier and Robert Gallo, who have admitted that there *never* was an HIV retrovirus or virus that could be identified![71]

"Up to today, there is no single scientifically convincing evidence for the existence of HIV. Not even one such a retrovirus has been isolated and purified by the methods of classical virology." Dr. Heinz Ludwig Sanger is an Emeritus Professor of Molecular Biology and Virology at the Max-Planck Institute for Biochemistry, Munich.[72]

Listen to this deception! In May 1983, doctors of the Institute Pasteur in France reported that they had isolated a new virus, which they suggested might cause AIDS... But, seven years later, "Dr. Ulrich Marcus, the press spokesman of the Robert Koch Institute reported that the HIV-virus cannot be isolated." District Court of Dortmund, Germany- Stefan Lanka and K. Krafeld, taken from the book "*Vaccination. Genocide in the Third Millennium?*" [73]

In 1984, Robert Gallo published four articles in *Science* (a scientific journal) along with others, *claiming* he had isolated HIV and concluded that it was the probable cause of AIDS. Several years later, *Robert Gallo*, HIV "discoverer," along with thirty-seven legal, medical, and research professionals, sent a letter to the journal *Science*, asking it to *officially retract* the original four papers making the case for HIV as the cause of AIDS. According to the letter's authors, *widespread evidence has now emerged that the studies were not only poorly carried out but that their results **were falsified**!!*

Along with a copy of the handwritten changes, the letter from the thirty-seven experts *includes* a letter from Robert Gallo himself, *admitting that HIV could not be isolated from human samples* alone, and a letter from an electron microscope expert saying that there was **"no HIV contained in Gallo's 1984 samples."**

Dr. Kary Mullis, Nobel Prize winner for the Polymerase chain reaction (PCR) test in 1993, states, *"If there is proof that HIV is the cause of AIDS, there should be scientific documents which either singly or collectively demonstrate that fact, at least with a high probability. There is no such document."* [74]

In 1996, *Luc Montagnier*, one of the other "discoverers" of HIV, admitted in the documentary *"AIDS-The Doubt,"* *"There is no scientific proof that HIV causes AIDS."*

Reinhard Kurth, director of the Robert Koch Institute, which is the leader in AIDS research, conceded in Der Speigel (September 9th, 2004), "*We don't exactly know how HIV causes disease.*" [75]

Walter Gilbert, Nobel Prize winner in microbiology at Harvard University, stated in 1989 that "he would not be surprised if there were another cause of AIDS and even that HIV was not involved." He also stated, "The major thing that concerns me by calling HIV the cause of AIDS IS THAT WE DO NOT HAVE PROOF OF CAUSATION." [76]

Dr. Stefan Lanka, an expert virologist, states, "No particle of HIV has ever been obtained pure, free of contaminants, nor has a complete piece of HIV RNA (or the transcribed DNA) ever been proved to exist."[77]

The largest and best-conceived study about sex and AIDS shows that AIDS is not a sexually transmitted disease! Nancy Padian's 1997 "Study on Seroconversion Rates Among Couples," in the Journal of American Medical Association, states, "the fact is glaringly obvious in the most comprehensive paper on this topic in it ***not a single case could be uncovered in which an HIV negative partner eventually became positive through sexual contact with his or her or HIV positive partner.***" That is to say, the observed transmission rate was zero.

Dr. Root-Bernstein is a physiologist at Michigan State University and the author of the book "*Rethinking AIDS.*" "When I look at AIDS patients, I can find that no one who develops AIDS does not have a multitude of immunosuppressant agents working on them simultaneously. The logic of the war on AIDS is seriously flawed."[78]

When he was asked what would happen if an otherwise healthy person was exposed to HIV, he said, "There are people who are married to blood transfusion patients, people who are married to hemophiliacs, who have been exposed to HIV from these means. There are surgeons who cut themselves all the time while working on AIDS patients, and all these people are free of HIV." Nothing would happen.[79]

A 1993 national TV special on mainstream television did a special feature, "What is the Real Cause of AIDS?" The show began by stating that HIV and AIDS have no proven correlation. It then switched to *the man with the deep pockets in the AIDS establishment*," Dr. Anthony Fauci. Dr. Fauci, then director of the National Institute of Allergy and Infectious Disease, said, "What's next is to develop an appropriate, safe, and effective therapy and a safe and effective vaccine. That's the bottom line of it. You have a disease, you identify the cause, you identify a treatment, and you get a vaccine for it."[80] Again, the ONLY OPTION he presented was to push a VACCINE! Ulterior motive, anyone??

Hmmm, do you hear anything familiar to the trillion-dollar COVID-19 vaccine agenda?

The AIDS symptoms in our country more likely stemmed from either fear of subsequent testing and treatments (www. learninggnm.com.)[81] or from "new" recreational drugs (like poppers or inhalants). These were "new" drugs with strong side effects used by many homosexuals.

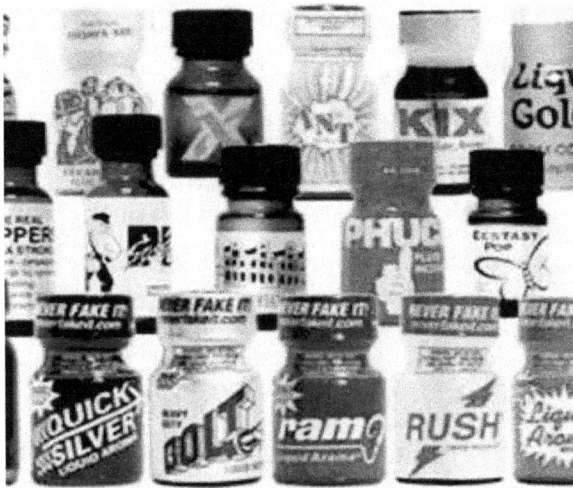

Poppers became very popular in the late 1970s. Sales added up to $50,000,000 in 1976 in just one state! "By 1977, poppers had permeated every angle of gay life, and in 1979, more than 5,000,000 people consumed poppers more than once a week." writes Harry Haverkos, who joined the CDC in 1981 and was the leading official during the AIDS movement.

Poppers have side effects known to severely damage the immune system, genes, lungs, liver, heart, and brain; they can produce neural damage similar to that of multiple sclerosis, or can have carcinogenic effects, and can lead to "sudden sniffing death." And the medical industry knew about its various dangers.

In 1981, the New England Journal of Medicine published several articles at the same time pointing out the use of drugs and the fast-lane lifestyle as possible causes of AIDS. Besides the widespread use of poppers and nitrate inhalants, this lifestyle often included many other toxic drugs. Those drugs include crystal meth, cocaine, crack, barbiturates, ecstasy, heroin, Librium, LSD Mandrex, MDA, MDM, mescaline, mushrooms, purple haze,

Seconal, special K, Tuinal, THC, PCP, STP, DMT, SDK, WDW, window pane, blotter, orange, sunshine, sweet pea, sky blue, Christmas tree dust, Benzedrine, Dexedrine, Dexamyl, Desoxyn, Clogidal, Nesperan, Tytch, nestex, black beauty, certyn, preludin with B12, zayl, quaalude, Nembutal, amytal, phenobarbital, Elavil, valium, Darvon, mandrax, opium, stidyl, halidax, caldfyn, optimal and drayl.[82]

The fast lane of the homosexual lifestyle often included a poor diet and long-term use of antibiotics and anti-fungal substances, which damage the mitochondria (and mitochondria are the bacterial powerhouses of the cells)!

The HIV scare started with five seriously ill gay men in 1981. Gottleib, a scientist from the University of California, brought these five men together after searching for several months to create a link between homosexuals and infectious diseases. The men had had no contact with each other; however, it was speculated that they had gotten ill from sexual contact. However, none of the men had sexual contact with anyone who was reported sick.

The CDC found in this "discovery" an *opportunity to create a whole new epidemic* since research funding for proving viruses caused cancer was soon running out. There was a widespread media message that caused the belief and panic that a deadly contagious sexually transmitted epidemic was occurring, at least among gay men. "Even though there was no scientific data to back up these perceptions. The CDC, the gay community, and the pharmaceutical companies were also behind in suppressing any information that drugs were causing AIDS.

Guess what? The CDC set on the search for a deadly virus and even tried to hide data. In 1982, the CDC's own AIDS expert, Harry Haverkos, analyzed three drugs, including poppers, and concluded that the drugs did play a weighty role in AIDS. However, the CDC refused to publish their own high-ranking employee's study. Haverkos transferred to the FDA in 1984 to become an AIDS coordinator there. In 1985, the paper finally appeared in the journal *Sexually Transmitted Diseases,* Haverkos, Harry, Disease Manifestation among Homosexual Men with Acquired Immunodeficiency Syndrome: A Possible Role of Nitrites in Kaposi's Sarcoma, *Sexually Transmitted Diseases*, October–December 1985.[83]

The Wall Street Journal published an article stating that ***drug abuse was so common among AIDS patients that this, and not the HIV virus, must be considered the primary cause of AIDS.*** [84]

In Africa, AIDS became a catch-all diagnosis for any number of symptoms common to many other diseases. Or better yet, there were many diseases linked to the term AIDS. There was no universal definition of AIDS (Acquired Immune Deficiency Syndrome). So, anyone suffering from many non-specific symptoms like weight loss, diarrhea, and itching was labeled an AIDS diagnosis. The HIV/AIDS epidemic is actually a smorgasbord of well-known diseases, many of which correlate closely with poverty. [85]

CHAPTER 29

What About All the Positive HIV Tests?

❦

The HIV antibody testing used for diagnosing HIV has some huge issues with false positives. Nobel Prize winner Kary Mullis, known for inventing the PCR test used for COVID-19, states, *"They got some big numbers for HIV-positive people in Africa before they realized that antibodies to malaria -which everyone in Africa has- shows up as HIV positive on tests."* [86] And not only Malaria but also dozens of other typical illnesses like chronic fever, weight loss, diarrhea, and tuberculosis *all* cause HIV-positive test results.

T-cells are "immune system" cells produced by the thymus. T-Cells can vary from day to day. One way doctors were flagrantly passing out AIDS diagnoses was to label anyone in Africa with a low T-cell count as an AIDS patient! Isn't that ludicrous?!

Max Essex, who is said to be one of the founding fathers of AIDS science, observed that lepers reacted positively to the HIV test. He pointed out that the results of the tests should be taken with a grain of salt.

The tragic consequences of an HIV-positive AIDS diagnosis meant that often African villagers were banished from their village to struggle with their illness alone. This often meant starvation and death.

Nevell Hodgkinson, a medical correspondent for the *Sunday Times,* spent weeks traveling through Africa. He says, "When I asked people what disease they were dying of, they replied: 'from AIDS,' whereupon I inquired: 'But from which disease in particular?' To this, they said: 'This patient has Tuberculosis, that one chronic diarrhea, this one Malaria, and that one Leprosy', all diseases that have been known in Africa for ages. But then everything was re-diagnosed as AIDS out of fear of AIDS." [87]

Dr. Peter Duesberg is a pioneering virologist at the University of California at Berkley. He said, "I would drink HIV-infested water all day long. There would be absolutely no risk in doing so. **There is no proof that HIV causes AIDS.** In addition, I am familiar with retroviruses, how they begin and what they do, and on those counts, I am confident enough that HIV, no matter how, couldn't cause AIDS." He says many researchers *know that truth* but can't afford to speak up. He states, "Many people tell me that they can't afford to speak up now because their research plans and grant money depend on HIV. (They say) If I join you, my grants will be terminated just like yours." [88]

CHAPTER 30

What Caused All the *Deaths* from AIDS?

❧

There were a number of different causes of AIDS depending on your location.

"AIDS is a combination of symptoms that existed already long before the invention of AIDS." Dr. Ryke Hamer, MD

The AZT (chemotherapy) treatments and other drugs used for AIDS, as well as the emotional shock and stress of the AIDS diagnosis given with a positive HIV test, were the cause of the majority of deaths.

Dr. Anthony Fauci, the most powerful AIDS official, refused to be interviewed regarding the lack of evidence that AZT had *any* positive outcome. Dr. Fauci has a long history of deception. *The "Fischl study" was the one study that was done to*

validate AZT, a known chemotherapy-like medication.
AZT proved extremely deadly to all the recipients in the
study.

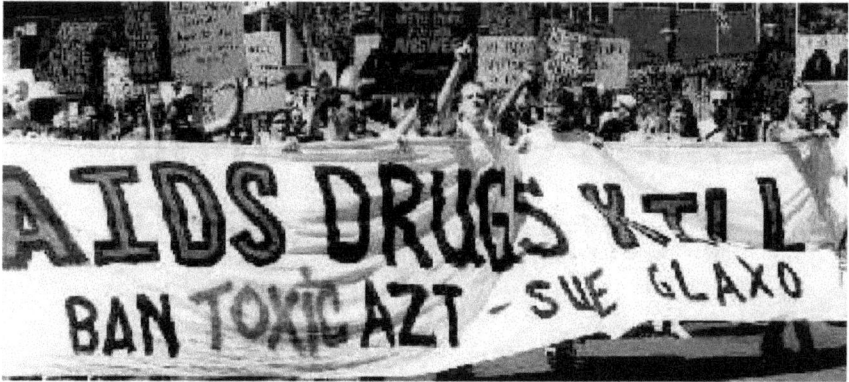

Basketball player Earvin "Magic" Johnson was one of the most famous survivors of the AZT prescription. He admits he took AZT for only a short time due to its horrible side effects. Thankfully, he never followed his doctor's advice, and he regained his health despite his HIV-positive diagnosis. He has been quoted as saying, "There is no magic in AZT, and there is no AZT in Magic." [89]

Unfortunately, the Russian Rudolf Nureyev, held by many to be the greatest ballet dancer of all time, also took AZT at the end of the 1980s. Nureyev was HIV positive, but otherwise, he was healthy. His personal physician, Dr. Michel Canesi, warned him about the deadly effects of AZT, but Nureyev was too scared to stop the drug. He died in 1993.

Sadly, famed tennis star Author Ashe followed his doctors' wishes. He never stopped his treatment despite saying that "standard treatments such as AZT actually make matters worse." He died at age 36.

Over 20 million people have died of an "AIDS" diagnosis and/or treatment. Many would contend that AIDS symptoms represent any number of toxins or illnesses that were present before the *invention* of AIDS. Patients were labeled as having AIDS when, in all reality, it could have been anything that caused a toxic reaction since every single symptom of AIDS is also that of toxicity.

The United Nations predicted that ninety million Africans would die of AIDS by 2025.

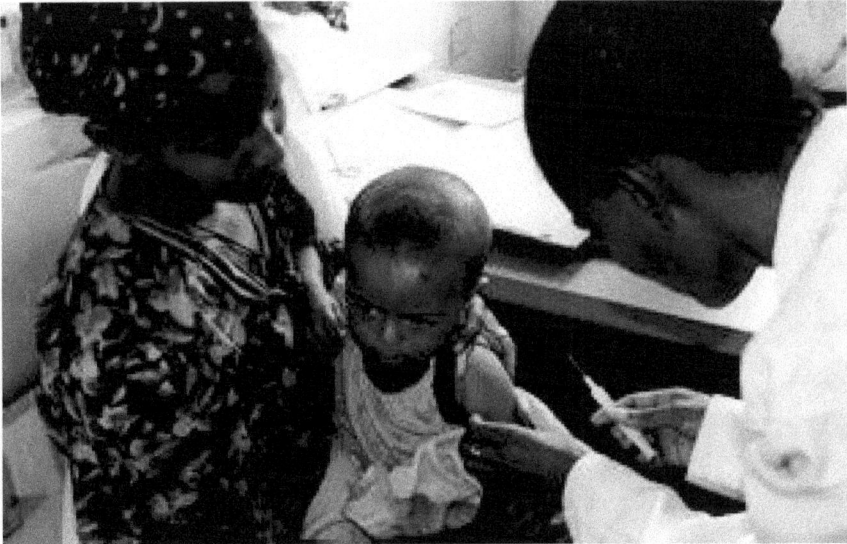

In Africa, the hepatitis B and smallpox vaccines were forced upon millions of unsuspecting Africans. These vaccines were full of toxins. When the populations exhibited AIDS symptoms after reacting to the toxins in the vaccines, they were given AZT. Death followed soon after the treatment.

On January 13, 2016, WHO actually *admitted* that the smallpox vaccine created AIDS/HIV in Africa.

CHAPTER 31

What's the Truth About the Coronavirus?

❧

"If you want to predict the future, invent it."

In October 2019, Event 201, a high-level pandemic "dress rehearsal" exercise, was conducted in case a pandemic broke out around the world. It was a collaborative effort between Dr. Fauci, the Johns Hopkins Center for Health Security, The World Economic Forum, and the Bill & Melinda Gates Foundation.

Event 201 included "...techniques for controlling official narratives, silencing dissent, forcibly masking large populations, and leveraging the pandemic to promote mandatory mass vaccinations."

The purpose of Event 201 was to simulate a hypothetical global pandemic caused by a novel *coronavirus*, exploring the potential impact on public health, economies, and international corporations.

NO KIDDING! LOOK IT UP!! An actual playbook meeting…

In December 2019, two months later, a "new" pandemic caused by a novel coronavirus was announced called Covid-19. It was said to have been started by a new highly contagious coronavirus called SAR-Cov-2 from Wuhan, China. Really? Event 201 was very prophetic. We need the eye-roll, wide-eyed, and/or throwing-up emoji here!

There are a number of common symptoms that are labeled as Covid-19. The list includes fever, cough, difficulty breathing, fatigue, body aches, headache, sore throat, loss of taste, loss of smell, congestion or runny nose, nausea or vomiting, diarrhea, or no symptoms at all. If the testing method involved a long nasal swab that was rubbed to clear up the nose of an individual (on their smell receptors and cribriform plate), wouldn't that alone irritate the nose and cause one to lose their sense of smell?

Interestingly, *every* Cold or Flu is comprised of the same list of possible symptoms. For example, the number of people who lost their sense of taste or smell during a cold or flu averaged about 14% *before* the introduction of COVID-19 in 2019. The people hospitalized for COVID-19 had an average of three other conditions, all likely to contribute to the above list of symptoms. In other words, the list of symptoms is nothing "new," and this is not a new "disease."

What was new about COVID-19 was the fear and propaganda that spread around the world because major media outlets are controlled by those who are making the most money (research Operation Mockingbird). More about how fear contributed to Covid-19 later.

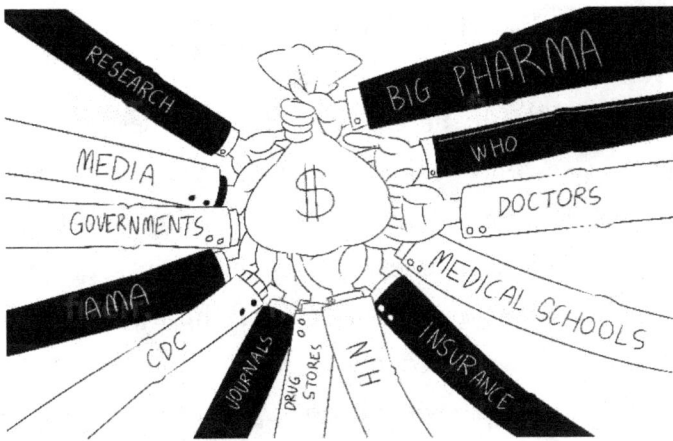

As mentioned earlier, with all colds and flu, the body goes through a "detox" process. As we go through our weeks and months of normal life, we build up toxins from what we think, feel, eat, drink, breathe, etc. This "toxic load" has to be released from the body at some point, so most people have a time during the year that they go through this toxic "unloading process." The symptoms of detoxing are your cold or flu. It typically happens in the late fall or spring, when the seasons are changing, or after the holidays. Just like nature goes through its own sort of detox when trees lose their leaves. The perfect time to announce a "new" disease would be the height of the normal cold and flu season.

According to the statistics, during COVID-19, there were no more Colds or Flus. **Everyone who had Cold or Flu symptoms (or no symptoms) after December 2019 was diagnosed with COVID-19!**

We now know from statistics that the official yearly death count for COVID-19 in 2020 or 2021 was the same as the flu in any other year previous. Covid-19 was not the deadly disease that propaganda would have you believe.

However, the fear created by Covid-19 was a perfect excuse to roll out vaccines and the new drug Remdesivir.

Even though both the vaccines and Remdesivir lacked any proof of safety or effectiveness, the public was introduced to the billion-dollar "solutions" to our "terrifying COVID-19 problem." The drug of choice, Remdesivir, was shown in some studies to cause complete organ failure in 30% of those participants who took the drug! It was used on most patients who entered the hospital after April 2020 with Covid-19 symptoms. It was used for 5-10 days with a whopping cost of $3100/patient. Combining that treatment with the ventilation masks (which actually created more difficulty breathing) and other drugs like the sedative Midazolam (which also caused respiratory difficulty) became a recipe for a higher death toll for patients who decided to go into the hospital or care facility.

According to the Medicare (CMS) data, 26% to 46% of those treated with Remdesivir *died* within 14 days of treatment. The number of deaths in the United States skyrocketed after the start of Remdesivir treatments in May 2020 as compared to those countries that did not use Remdesivir.

And what was another unusual aspect of the profitable pandemic? There was a government pay-out for every death recorded as Covid-19. Every diagnosed death was worth over $30,000 to a hospital. Hospital administrators were incentivized to have deaths occur from anyone diagnosed with COVID-19! In other words, it was very profitable to have a patient die!!

You may have heard of a friend of a friend who died in a motorcycle accident that was labeled Covid-19. A study published in the journal *Clinical Infectious Diseases* and other CDC data both conclude that 30% of the official COVID-19 death toll includes people who had a different underlying cause of death.

So why would it be important to increase the statistical number of cases and deaths from Covid-19? If you want people to do something, the best way is to create fear. Studies show that fear induces a lack of logical thinking (common sense). And what was the purpose of promoting fear? You probably guessed it: money. Money from the sale of the solution to our fear... Vaccines. Along with the wealth that was shifted from the small businesses (that were shut down around the world) to the large corporations.

The 100 research studies that showed that inexpensive treatments like hydroxychloroquine and ivermectin could reduce symptoms and shorten the illness were simply ignored because they weren't part of the agenda.

After all, they had already practiced the playbook in EVENT 201. They had a plan and a purpose for Covid-19. Now you know why people have been saying "Plandemic"!

On December 16, 2019, Moderna brought their finished coronavirus vaccine to the University of North Carolina. Previously, Moderna was a bankrupt company that had never made a drug or a vaccine. You might wonder what kind of crystal ball helped Moderna out. War games and dress rehearsals!

In 2018, millions of dollars were spent on COVID-19 Diagnostic Test instruments and apparatus kits. The EU, Denmark, United States, Uruguay, Germany, Japan, and Singapore all had large purchases two years before the official "outbreak." [90]

It seems as if all the countries are getting ready for a big pandemic.

CHAPTER 32

So, What Was the Coronavirus That Scientists Were "Seeing"?

Let's look at Rivers' Postulates, which are again used as the gold standard to prove that a virus causes a disease.

Rivers' Postulates are:

1. The virus can be isolated from a diseased organism.
2. The virus can be cultivated and made to grow cells of a new organism.
3. Proof of filterability—the virus can be separated from a medium that also contains bacteria.
4. The filtered virus will produce a comparable disease when the cultivated virus is used to infect experimental animals.
5. The virus can be re-isolated from the infected experimental animal.
6. A specific immune response to the virus can be detected.[91]

Although Rivers' postulates were expanded, to this day, NO DISEASE HAS EVER BEEN PROVEN WITH THEM! Even though these are the "gold standard," and they make sense to all scientists, we'll repeat NO DISEASE HAS EVER BEEN PROVEN WITH THEM (including coronavirus)!

The steps that scientists have taken to isolate a coronavirus are as follows. We'll let **YOU** determine how isolated this can be.[92]

1. Take a spit sample from a sick patient with a cough.
2. Centrifuge and take the cellular part (which supposedly has the virus) and leave the liquid.
3. This is called "purification"!! This goop of centrifuged cells.
4. Take this "purification" of God-only-knows-what and add it to monkey kidney cells.
5. Grow this concoction until there is enough cellular material to work with.
6. Centrifuge again and examine under an electron microscope.

Seriously? Is this the virus isolation method used? If you read this, you can see how there is **NO WAY** they would know if what they are looking at came from the cells of the animal or the cells of the patient! Plus, they don't have a purified or isolated virus in any sense of the word!

Another research study that researchers have used as "proof" that a *coronavirus causes a disease* is:

1. Take the nose mucus of sick people.
2. Grow this snot with a mixture of *monkey kidney cells.*

3. Centrifuge this crazy mixture.

4. Inject this "purification" of cellular mix into two monkeys.

One monkey developed whooping cough, and the other had some sort of respiratory symptoms from the snot/kidney cell mixture they called a coronavirus "purification." And that, my friend, is so-called "proof" that a "coronavirus" causes disease! Can you see how anything in the mixture could cause the symptoms? There is absolutely nothing isolated or purified at all.

No study has proven that *coronavirus*, or *any virus*, is disease-causing or contagious, nor has any study proven anything except that the Germ Theory is false!

Even the head of the Chinese CDC said the virus was not isolated when he was asked by NBC Nightly News why they didn't share information with the US regarding the coronavirus and its threat to public health. Dr. Wu Zunyou said, **"They didn't isolate the virus, that's the problem."** [93] And why not? *Because the virus isn't the cause of anything, and they can't isolate it and prove that it is!*

Dr. Andrew Kaufman, MD, is a well-known researcher of viruses and truth. He has a great question-and-answer website we would highly recommend![94]

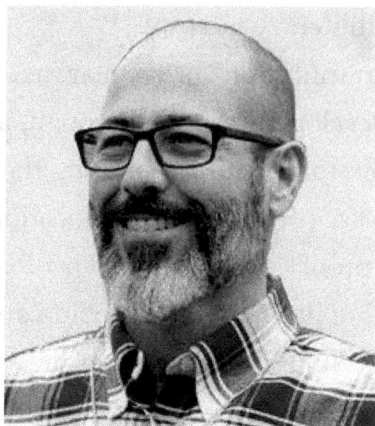

andrew@andrewkaufmanmd.com

When we were first doing our research about viruses, we came across a YouTube video by Dr. Andrew Kaufman, MD, in early 2020. Since that time, Dr. Kaufman has been very instrumental and courageous in educating the masses on the truth of viruses, Covid-19, and Germ Theory. He and his team have done hundreds, if not thousands, of hours of research to find out the truth about the disease.

CHAPTER 33

Spider-Man and Snipe Hunting

❧

Why do they have so many pictures of the coronavirus? Because they have *talented graphics artists* and *computer-generated images* that make wonderful artwork.

Do you like Spider-Man movies? Millions of people do. And millions of people know that most images in movies are made with computer-generated imagery (CGI). However, when the movie is over, everyone knows that it is pure "make-believe." Right! Spider-Man does not exist in real life. Are we so conditioned to think anything we see on the internet or in the media is inherently real?

An electron microscope cannot be used to look at anything living, and the images are *always grainy black and white*. Thus, there is no evidence that the virus is entering the cell or "infecting" it, and the color images are all graphics. The live images from the atomic force microscope research prove that the viruses (exosomes) are *leaving* the cell to help it.

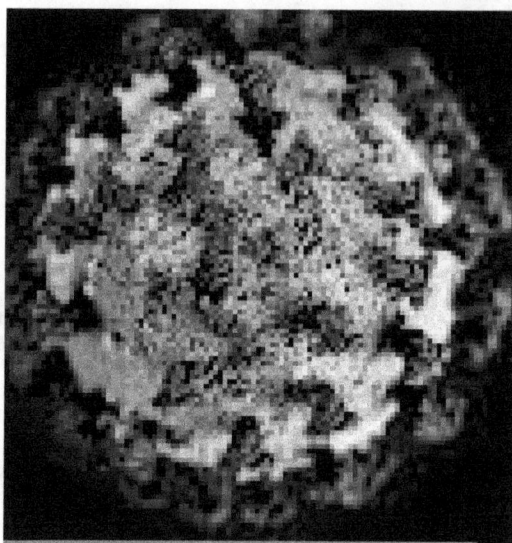

Computer graphic

A virus isn't the cause of anything, and they can't isolate it and prove that it is!! If you study the research, it is computer-generated pictures in fancy words. It's the trickery of CGI and a scary "you could die" diagnosis that literally scares the "breath out of us" along with ulterior motives to sell the public on drugs and vaccines. The diagnosis *itself* is a biological shock/conflict, and innocent people unknowingly start down the path of a Significant Biological Program (SBP). Whether the coronavirus had ever been isolated has been challenged in court many times, and each time, the ruling states that the coronavirus has NEVER been isolated!

As far as contagion studies are concerned, there are not any that prove contagion but rather the OPPOSITE! You can look at your own experience. We all know someone who said they had the COVID-19 virus or tested positive, and their spouse or family members had no issues. Rarely do any of us even know of anyone who died unless they were old or sick. We all know someone who felt VERY toxic with something they called COVID-19. So, yes, there were toxins.

Labs cannot "make a virus," the only thing they can do is put together genetic coding strands to produce a protein. They cannot genetically change a virus due to the fact they can't even isolate one! Another important thing to remember, as you frantically clean your hands and surfaces to "kill" a virus, is that _viruses aren't living_! They are non-living nano particulates that are mRNA or part DNA strands surrounded by a protein, and THEY ARE NOT ALIVE. That means viruses don't move, they don't replicate, and they don't fly. They don't inject themselves into a cell to "infect" it. Viruses are already "harmlessly" in your cells. They don't fly around in your spit or breath, and they don't "live" on surfaces for any length of time.

The collective Big Pharma and medical government institutions remind us of a game called "Snipe Hunting." Do you know what a "Snipe" is? Young adolescents like the challenge of hunting for "Snipes" in the dark of night. You can picture young male adolescents holding a burlap sack and running as fast they can through trees and brush to catch as many "Snipes" as they can snag. The boys can't wait to _brag_ about how many they caught the following day. Guess what? The "Snipes" are fictitious creatures! You could hunt as many as you want and claim _more_ than you bagged!

It sounds like what some virologists at the CDC have fed the public about viruses. It's time that we should stop falling for their deceptions. Why should anyone believe the CDC when they are self-governed and self-regulated? They can say whatever they think is "highly probable" and "most likely" all they want with all the taxpayer money they receive, but why would you believe them?

Why *should* you believe them? We know it's human nature not to want to feel like you have been deceived. In this book, we are giving you the knowledge and power to start *THINKING FOR YOURSELF!*

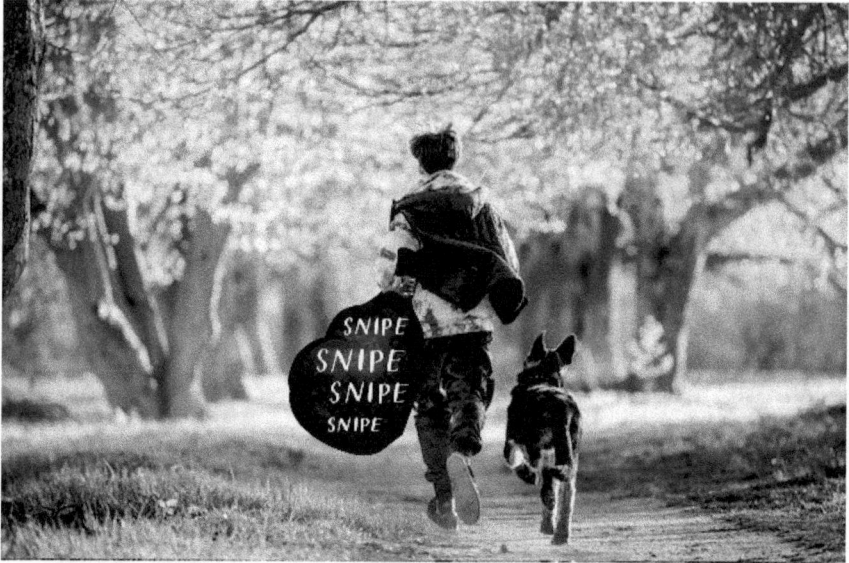

The WHO, CDC, NIH, and Dr. Fauci are all under investigation for their part in creating a huge epidemic scare with no scientific proof. The total mortality rate and risk come up at less than a normal flu year.

The bottom line is that you cannot breathe on someone and kill them. You can't hug someone or shake their hand and harm them with any germ or virus. That is a man-made fairy tale that has no basis in the scientific method!

Mother Nature, God, Divine, whatever label you want to use, has a higher plan than to make us fear each other because of a "deadly" virus. We are told biblically *not* to fear. Fear is used as a propaganda tool for money-making purposes. The news media is used as a tool for profit. The false Germ Theory is used for profits.

Let's let go of our fear and use our common sense. Someone once said, "If it doesn't make sense, it's a LIE!"

Yes, you or your friend may have come down with some flu-like symptoms. That simply means you were "highly toxic" with something your body really didn't like and needed to purge. Or you or your friend "expected" to come down with something because of all the fear-mongering media, and so you did (nocebo-effect). Or there were literally people who were "scared to death."

Sometimes, when we face a threat to our survival that can come from a pandemic scare, a cancer diagnosis, or even the headlines in the news media, our brain reacts like it's been hit with a "Voodoo Spell," and all we can think of is "How long do I have to live?" We could experience a "death fright scare" conflict in the terms of German New Medicine and start down the road of what we label a disease.

Just like the study of the Laos men in the book "*The Expectation Effect*," our fear can be so strong that it can induce death.

And, yes, people died with flu-like symptoms. But now we know...**the COVID-19 pandemic, according to the stats, was about as deadly as the normal flu in any given year, and numbers were inflated because practically everyone who died in 2020-2022 was labeled a COVID-19 death.**

Honestly, we are completely and utterly filled with viruses. It ISN'T even logical that they are evil, infectious particles. Yes, the computer "virus" infects your computer and messes with your information, but you are not your computer! You CANNOT be hacked!! Your common sense can be hacked by the media and pharmaceutical companies that sell vaccines. But that is about it. Together, we can put an end to the MASS DECEPTION!

"COVID-19 is not the problem; it is a problem, one largely solvable with early treatments that are safe, effective, and inexpensive. The problem is endemic corruption in the medical industrial complex, currently supported at every turn by mass media companies. This cartel's coup d'état has already siphoned billions from taxpayers, already vacuumed up trillions from the global middle class, and created the excuse for massive propaganda, censorship, and control worldwide. Along with its captured regulators, this cartel has ushered in the global war on freedom and democracy." - Robert F. Kennedy Jr. from *"The Real Anthony Fauci"* [95]

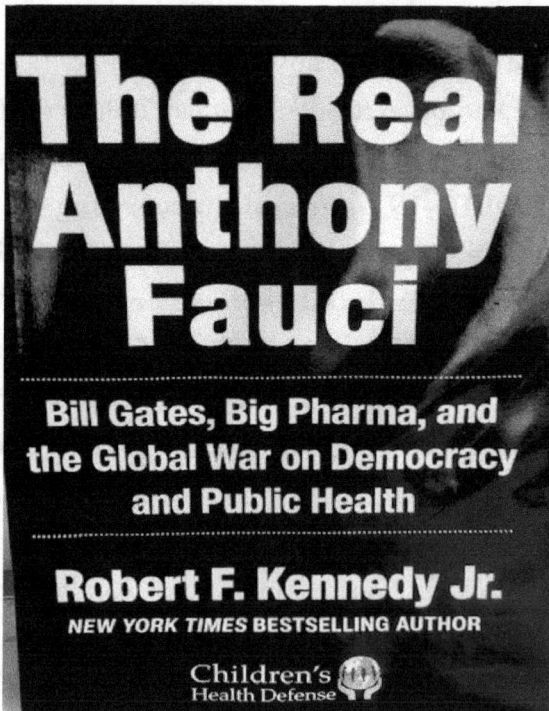

The Real Anthony Fauci

Bill Gates, Big Pharma, and the Global War on Democracy and Public Health

Robert F. Kennedy Jr.
NEW YORK TIMES BESTSELLING AUTHOR

Children's
Health Defense

CHAPTER 34

What About the PCR Tests?

❧

"Scientists are doing an awful lot of damage to the world in the name of helping it. I don't mind attacking my own fraternity because I am ashamed of it." - Dr. Kari Mullis

The PCR Test is adjustable to test positive for whatever antibody a doctor wants to detect. One could adjust the PCR test and "tune it in" to detect the antibodies of your tears: It was used as the "gold standard" to diagnose Covid-19 and for statistical data related to cases and deaths. But what did its inventor, Kary Mullis, have to say about it? **"You cannot use the PCR test to prove causation from a virus and it cannot be used to diagnose illness."** What was that? Was he trying to warn us that the test should not be used as a deceptive tactic for any other agenda?

Dr. Kary Mullis (1944-2019) won the Nobel Prize in Chemistry in 1993 for the creation of the Polymerase Chain Reaction (PCR) test. He was a brilliant scientist who, for years, was one of Dr. Anthony Fauci's biggest critics. Dr. Fauci is the head of the National Institute of Allergy and Infectious Disease (NIAID) and has a big influence on the National Institute of Health (NIH), which makes a lot of US Health policy decisions. He worked parallel to Dr. Fauci during the AIDS pandemic in the 1990s. Mullis said, "Guys like Fauci get up there and start talking, and you know he doesn't know anything really about anything, and I'd say that to his face. Nothing. The man thinks you can take a blood sample and stick it in an electron microscope, and if it's got a virus in there, you'll know it... He doesn't understand electron microscopy and he doesn't understand medicine. And he should not be in the position he is in..." [96]

Do you suppose that there's a coincidence to his death in August of 2019, right before the announcement of the coronavirus? His official cause of death was "labeled" Whooping Cough, but it seems way too convenient that this outspoken scientist would be silenced right before the start of the hugest profit grab in our century.

It's been quite apparent from the many quotes attributed to Dr. Mullis that he was a huge critic of Dr. Fauci and would have publicly protested using his test for *diagnosing* the coronavirus.

The PCR Test was invented to be used for *research* to amplify a genetic sequence. It is a research tool only. In order for scientists to "see" a DNA sequence, they "amplify" it. When using it for COVID-19, the test could be *manipulated* to make any positive diagnosis for the coronavirus. The same was done in the HIV/

AIDs scare of the 1990s. The PCR Test was used to make the HIV diagnosis, and subsequently, millions of false HIV diagnoses were given. This diagnosis led to millions of deaths from the AZT treatment and fear.

PCR tests, Antibody tests, and every other test used for a coronavirus are surrogate tests. This means they have NEVER been compared to any "gold standard." If you don't have a *definitive* negative test or a *definitive* positive test to compare a test to, then all positive or negative results are USELESS. In other words, you must have a case that shows a definite positive that you can use to compare your test to from the beginning so you can "test" the accuracy of your test. This was never done. This, along with the fact that it was to be used only for research, makes the PCR Test completely useless.

As the inventor of the PCR test, Kary Mullis, tells us again and again, even back with HIV, "A PCR test should *never* be a tool in the *diagnosis of infectious diseases*." [97] Every package on a PCR Test has this statement printed on it!

Several world leaders questioned the PCR Test. One such leader was the president of Tanzania, Africa, named John Magufuli. President Magufuli said fruit and goats tested positive for COVID-19 when the tests were sent secretly to a lab. Apparently, he didn't trust the test as much as the rest of the world leaders. President Magufuli died of a cardiac arrest shortly after making those revelations public! Does his death sound suspicious?

A file from March 30, 2020, from the CDC and the FDA concedes: "Detection of viral RNA may not indicate the presence of an infectious virus or that 2019-nCoV is the causative agent for clinical symptoms" and "This test cannot rule out diseases caused by other bacterial or viral pathogens." So why has this test been used so extensively to determine how many deaths and cases there are from the pandemic?

FDA said, "Positive results do not rule out bacterial infection or co-infection with other viruses. The agent detected may not be the definite cause of disease."

Light Mix Modular SARS-CoV Assays are another test used. Here's their announcement, "These *assays are NOT intended for use as an aid in the diagnosis or coronavirus infection.*"

Seriously? Using those tests makes as much sense as being required to wear "protective" masks that come from a box that reads, "*These masks do not protect against the spread of infectious diseases.*" Did you get that? That is what we were mandated to do! Yet, they advertise that they don't protect you *right* on the boxes!

Clearly, if the test for the coronavirus is inaccurate and misleading, as is the case, and one can NOT prove that the coronavirus is the cause of COVID-19, then there aren't any grounds for believing the reports about the number of COVID-19 cases, the number of Covid-19 deaths, or any other statistics coming from the medical institutions.

CHAPTER 35

What's the Word on COVID-19 Contagion?

❧

The only thing contagious is the emotional shock that families or nations may face together, as in stress, tension, fear, or arguments. They also may face the same toxicity in their environment in man-made chemicals, mass vaccinations, Electrical Magnetic Frequencies (EMF), man-made food, air pollution (like glyphosate insecticides and chemtrails), and unclean water.

You can be sleeping near your spouse, children, or relatives who are sick, and often you don't get sick. You've heard of someone who's tested positive for coronavirus, and they made no one else sick even though they were quarantined together. Yes, people in the same family or at the same job sometimes get sick at the same time. And that's because they are experiencing the same toxins or life stresses at the same time. So, the body's response is *to get flu-like symptoms or cold symptoms to get rid of the toxins* through the lungs, urine, poop or skin. How amazing is your body! It's always working to keep you healthy!! Even when we toxify it repeatedly.

So, if there are no studies showing that you can catch anything, either bacterial, viral, or fungal, why don't they do some more? Because you can't catch anything! Remember the long list of disgusting contagion studies we mentioned in an earlier chapter that resulted in no one getting sick? Research will rarely be funded unless someone is going to benefit monetarily from that research.

No virus, bacteria, or fungi is contagious from another person. Not breathing on you. Not hugging. Not kissing. Not coughing. Not even having sex! These diseases you can think of all have a scientific explanation that starts with a toxin, either spiritual, mental, emotional, physical, or chemical!!

There are toxins in the air like EMFs or air pollutants, in the environment, on surfaces, in the water, in the food, in your body, thoughts, or emotions... there are toxins everywhere. But toxins, germs, and viruses are different.

The so-called coronavirus didn't fly around and TRY to kill you or make you sick. Toxins cannot be avoided, and toxic events cannot be avoided. But they can be identified and dealt with before they turn into a dis-ease. This is why there are many things on the planet that nature provides for us to remove the toxins from our bodies. One of the best ways to stay healthy is to recognize when something toxic has occurred to our psyche or our physical body. **Cleansing toxins (detoxing) spiritually (i.e., forgiveness), mentally (i.e., letting go of bad memories), emotionally (i.e., releasing anger), and physically (i.e., fasting or doing an intestinal cleanse) is key to being healthy!**

CHAPTER 36

Antibodies and COVID-19?

❧

The Antibody Theory says that before we encounter a virus or get sick from a virus, we have no antibodies to it. After getting sick, we develop specific antibodies to the specific "threat." Here's the problem with that theory: ***it has no consistency***, and it changes depending on the week. Also, have you noticed all the rules changed with this virus? You can be sick and have no antibodies, and you can be asymptomatic and be positive with antibodies. You can be negative and symptomatic. It's just a matter of what's needed for the desired outcome. In other words, there is no science to it at all!

Remember when scientists used to tell you that you couldn't get a viral disease again once you had it due to your antibodies? Why did they stop? We guess that nonsense didn't fit their agenda of wanting to vaccinate you repeatedly.

Antibodies are proteins, and they support your body when it is removing toxins and repairing, but *no scientific study shows they increase or decrease with a virus. Now THAT is big. No study shows antibodies increase or decrease with a virus.* They increase when you have been injected with something toxic! They increase when you have become toxic.

As for the production of antibodies and the immune system, here are the results from one huge study, "**Immunity is a grand medical delusion**... In 1950, the British Medical Society conducted *exhaustive studies* on the relationship between the incidence of diphtheria and the presence of antibodies. Their conclusion: **there is absolutely no relation between the two**." [98]

So, there you have it, an extensive study, and they found NO LINK and NO RELATION between antibodies and germs, bacteria, or viruses.

Antibodies, along with white blood cells and microorganisms, are involved in wound healing, cellular repair, and clearing toxins. However, their presence is not linked to any specific germ. **There are absolutely no tests that indicate that antibodies are specific to anything!**

CHAPTER 37

What's the Deal With All the Vaccines? They're Working, Right?

❧

We often come across the philosophical debates that ensue about vaccines. We call it philosophical, but it could also be termed *religious*. There is blind faith so many people have in the power of vaccines to help their families stay healthy. People believe in their doctors and the so-called "science" of the safety studies and the "dangers" of not being vaccinated.

Often, it is best to stay quiet and pretend you agree. No one wants to be labeled the dreaded "anti-vaxxer." The label is nothing short of being murderous and idiotic simultaneously. However, we can't even express the heartbreak that we have over the hundreds of people we know who have been affected by vaccine injury.

In the health profession, we hear our fair share of stories from taking the histories of patients. Still, the vaccine industry has a

VERY good storyline they put on across all the media platforms based on the germ theory only. And once you know the secret of the germ theory fraud, the contagion fraud, and even the epidemic fraud, we hope you can consider the rest of these facts when you're making your future health decisions.

C H A P T E R   3 8

Christine's Story

❧

Let us tell you the heartbreaking story of Christine, who lost her daughter after being vaccinated. She writes, *"Death from vaccination is neither quick nor painless. I helplessly watched my daughter suffer an excruciatingly slow death as she screamed and arched her back in pain while the vaccine assaulted her immature immune system. The poisons used as preventatives seeped through her tiny body, overwhelming her vital organs one by one until they collapsed... My beautiful, innocent, infant daughter, death by lethal injection."* - Christine C. (her daughter died 24 hours after receiving a DPT shot.)

The real story began 150 years ago...

The idea behind vaccines was started in the 1800s. It's defined as producing Immunity to a disease caused by a virus by using a "special preparation" to stimulate the production of appropriate antibodies. Therein lies the problem. *The vaccine "preparation" is always a mixture of horribly toxic substances to stimulate a reaction.* Usually, the *reaction* is sickness. Initially, it was often death! Remember, we discovered in the private notes of Louis Pasteur that ALL of his vaccine experiments were failures, resulting in death.

CHAPTER 39

We Have All Heard That Vaccines Save Millions of Lives

Does vaccination save lives? Nothing could be further from the truth. We'll give you a brief history of the disaster that started as "inoculations." In 1796, pus from cows was used in inoculations to "prevent disease." Originally, pus from oozing cowpox sores was mixed with the blood of a healthy individual and injected to create "freedom from disease." Although many died from this procedure and there were increased rates of smallpox in towns that used this procedure, it was used until 1840. Finally, "inoculations" were deemed too deadly! They were discontinued due to the large number of smallpox cases *after inoculations* were given!

"As a rule, a certain percentage of fatalities and the contagiousness of the inoculated cases made the practice hazardous. Inoculation was prohibited in England in 1840." [99]

And then, as profiteering science would have it ...Along came the famous Edward Jenner.

Edward Jenner is regarded by the medical industry as a hero (ironically) for *his* smallpox vaccine. He got his idea from the same inoculation myth told by milkmaids that if you injected the pus from cows inflicted with cowpox, humans would have a less severe case of smallpox. He used this mixture without doing any known scientific experiments and was paid very well.

Although Jenner is often called a physician, it is documented that he did not study for or pass the medical exam but purchased his medical degree. His qualification as a fellow of the Royal Society of England was not a result of any work related to medical matters but rather of the results of his study on the life of the *cuckoo bird!*

The only paper about vaccination that Jenner submitted to the Royal Society was rejected because it lacked proof. Other than his rejected paper, no further scientific work was submitted by Edward Jenner to the Royal Society for approval on vaccination.

Herbert Shelton explains: "Neither Jenner nor any of his successors ever re-presented the claims for this vaccine, together with proofs to the Royal Society of England." But apparently, *belief in the cuckoo expert* was enough to roll out the vaccines.

In 1857, 17 years *after* the same deadly concoction was banned for causing smallpox (with no research), Edward Jenner got smallpox "inoculations" back out into the public with the new name "Vaccinations." You must wonder, considering the year, whether he knew much of Louis Pasteur. However, it wasn't until the end of that century that Pasteur would also contribute the harmful but profitable Rabies and Anthrax vaccines to an unsuspecting public.

So, what caused Smallpox, and why did it disappear?

CHAPTER 40

Smallpox and the Medical Hippocratic Oath of "First Do No Harm?"

Smallpox is an acute disease that causes a fever and a rash that scars the skin. It is said to be a bacterial disease, but we now know it is caused by toxic conditions associated with poverty, like poor sanitation, hygiene, and malnutrition. The medical establishment claims to have successfully eradicated this disease between the 1960s and 70s. However, history reveals that smallpox resided in cities due to overcrowding and sanitation issues. *It had nothing to do with the medical industry and vaccinations. As soon as hygiene and sanitation were implemented, smallpox disappeared.* Two cities, Cleveland, Ohio, and Leicester, England, both claim they became virtually free of smallpox by *abolishing vaccination* and increasing sanitation.

On the WHO website, it is quoted about the smallpox vaccine, "no government gives or recommends smallpox vaccine routinely since it *can cause serious complications and even death.*"

When mandatory smallpox *vaccines were required* in 1867, there *were 57,016 smallpox deaths* between the years of 1871 and 1880. When vaccinations *were discontinued,* the total death rate from smallpox disease between 1911 and 1920 numbered only *110 total deaths.*

So much for smallpox vaccinations eradicating the disease of smallpox, the only true eradication comes from eradicating the vaccine! How did we get so deceived about smallpox and vaccines? Propaganda and the medical industry "education."

CHAPTER 41

Goodbye Vaccinations!

❦

In his incredible book, *"Good-bye Germ Theory,"* Dr. William Trebing has extensive research available to anyone. Here is the book briefly and some of his findings regarding vaccines based on his research findings.[100]

Good-bye Germ Theory, Dr. William Trebing

- "Smallpox would never have been the problem it was if the smallpox vaccine was not invented and promoted. In populations where there was no vaccine there was no smallpox." - Glen Dettman, MD
- "Autism has increased by over 3000 times since the advent of mandatory vaccination programs, when it was considered very rare. The medical profession blames this on new diagnostic parameters, but this one cannot possibly have created such a drastic increase in so little time. The systematic blood poisoning of America's children through

mercury and other products in vaccines is the only event which could possibly do this."

- "Following mandatory vaccine programs one of every 149 children in Brick Township, NJ is autistic."

- "Following mandatory vaccine programs between 1993 and 1998, autism increased 513% in the state of Maryland."

- "In India, between the years of 2010 and 2017, there have been over 490,000 children who have been paralyzed due to the oral polio vaccine! This fact was confirmed by two leading doctors in two reputable hospitals. Despite the government-certified eradication of polio in India in 2011, the oral vaccine was given to millions of children by the Bill and Melinda Gates Foundation. -reported in the newspaper, The Hindu, "Vaccine-induced paralysis calls for action, says the study," by Bindu Shajan Perappandan.

- "Also, studies from Finland and Turkey suggest that Guillain-Barré Syndrome (GBS) is causatively associated with Oral Polio vaccination campaigns."

- "Doctors are instructed by the American Medical Association to downplay parents' concerns of vaccine reactions, and they deny any correlation of adverse reaction to vaccines they have just administered."

- "Federal government reports confirm the vaccinations kill more than three children per week in America."

- "Jonas Salk, creator of the famous Salk polio vaccine made a public statement in 1976 that 2/3 of the cases of polio which occurred between 1966 and 1976 were caused by his vaccine."

- "The DPT shot has been banned in most of Europe and Japan since 1975 due to its extreme toxicity, but American children still receive this vaccine."
- "Records prove the death rates from polio, pertussis, whooping cough and measles were decreasing on their own before the vaccines were introduced, and that present records were altered to demonstrate the decrease was due to vaccines."
- "Each year, they are approximately 950 deaths from the whooping cough vaccine as compared to 10 deaths from the actual disease."
- "Drug companies use the same pertussis shot to intentionally create encephalitis in experimental lab animals."
- "Over 95% of people who actually acquire diseases have been vaccinated *against* those very diseases! Drug companies refuse to study unvaccinated populations."
- "The "germ theory" does not follow any scientific guidelines to prove its validity. When assessed by the simple scientific method type in *elementary schools* it is proven invalid."
- "Pasteur's major credits do not belong to him but to another brilliant scientist called Pierre Bechamp, who totally disagreed with Pasteur's "germ theory" of disease creation. Most of Pasteur's early vaccine work ended in disaster."
- "The Center for Disease Control (CDC) charters an *epidemic intelligent service* which travels the country in search of symptoms they can use to formulate epidemics for profit! How disgusting is that?"

- "Most vaccination laws are completely unconstitutional and have no relevance to today's world. Local health departments promote most vaccine programs to acquire federal aid and grant money at the expense of America's children."

- "Everyone who wishes can enter a courtroom without the high cost of a lawyer, and WIN! You do not need to have to be vaccinated or to have your children vaccinated against your will."

- "The FDA has reported the doctors *under* report vaccine reactions by 90%."

- "In any given population, the majority people who become ill are those who are vaccinated."

- "Unvaccinated populations can be proven scientifically and otherwise far healthier than vaccinated ones."

- "Encephalitis (brain damage due to the swelling in the brain tissue) is an almost given side effect of vaccine toxins according to most research studies on vaccine damages."

- "15 to 20% of American school children are considered to be learning disabled with brain damage dysfunction directly caused by vaccines."

- "Your government has paid over 4 billion in vaccination damage claims."

- "Your child is 94 times more likely to die from a whooping cough vaccine them from the actual whooping cough and nearly 4000 times more likely acquiring long-term damage from the vaccine then from developing the disease."

- "The CDC is aware that Thimerosal (Mercury preservative in vaccines) is linked to autism by virtue of their own private research. However, they refused to provide the raw data from the studies, as requested by Congressman Dan Burton, to be used for an independent review by third-party research organization."

- "Giving a 10-pound infant a single vaccine in a day is the equivalent of giving 100-pound adult 40 vaccines in a day!"

- "Considering the above information, medical doctors insist on injecting 45 vaccines directly into your child's bloodstream by age 6 months; 64 by age 18 months; and 74 by age 6."

- "The CDC has an advisory committee on immunization practices called the ACIP. This committee advise lawmakers as to which vaccine should be mandated. ACIP is riddled with conflicts of interest, since committee members own patents for vaccines and stock in the pharmaceutical companies which make the vaccines."

- "Americans are amongst the most vaccinated people in the history of the planet and are also amongst the sickest in its history. 50% of all Americans suffer with at least one chronic disease, and 20% have 2 or more. These chronic diseases cause 70% of all American deaths."

- In 1986, the government passed a law to protect vaccine manufacturers from lawsuits regarding any vaccine-related injuries, giving them complete financial protection from any wrongdoing or safety issues.[101]

Turtles All The Way Down – Vaccine Science and Myth

- Clinical trials of vaccines are rigged to hide their true (and high) rate of side effects, which means the medical establishment's long-standing claim that vaccines are safe has no scientific merit.[102]

- Vaccine trials, in general, and childhood vaccine trials, specifically, are purposely designed to obscure the true incidents of adverse events of the vaccine being tested.[103]

- The rate of adverse events of the tested vaccine is said to be similar to the "background rate." Hence, it is considered safe. The researchers and the vaccine manufacturer they work for seem to "forget" that the compound they administered to the control group is a bioactive substance, carrying its own risks and side effects, and hardly represents the baseline or background rate that is essential to an RCT [Random Controlled Trial] for a new vaccine. Thus, the vaccine is approved and added to national vaccine programs throughout the world. Then, when the "next generation" vaccine comes along, its pre-licensing clinical trials will always compare the new vaccine to the current vaccine and never to a placebo. Thus, all parties involved ensure that the true rate of vaccine adverse events is never disclosed - for either the original or upgraded vaccine - and the rate is never shared with the public or even the medical world.[104]

- …this method is exactly the one vaccine manufacturers employ to deliberately obscure the real incidents of vaccine adverse events. The entire vaccine program is founded upon this deception.[105]

- ... The safety of GSK's 5-in-1 and 4-in-1 vaccines was tested against the triple vaccine (DTaP), which was tested against the older generation vaccine (DTP), whose safety was never tested in an RCT with a placebo control group. A turtle was standing on the back of a turtle, standing on the back of yet another turtle - all the way down.[106]

- ... none of the many products in either of the DTaP vaccine family lines routinely administered in the US has been tested for safety in a clinical trial with a placebo-controlled group.[107]

- Similar to MMR II, the original MMR was tested in a few small-to-medium trials, where the newer vaccine was given to a total of more than 1000 infants and children. The control groups' subjects totaled about 1/10 of that number, and most of them were siblings of the vaccinated children (which violates the randomization principle). The control group participants received no injection at all, which means the studies were not blinded; everyone knew who got the vaccine and who didn't. As with MMR II, the MMR trials fail to meet the Phase 3 RCT bar.

- Evidently, the safety of the MMR line of vaccines, like the rest of the vaccines in the US childhood vaccination program, was tested according to the de facto industry rule of "turtles all the way down." [108]

- ...tens of thousands of infants were given an utterly useless compound whose safety was unknown and whose side effects could be (and probably were in some cases) severe and permanent. Thus, the Phase 3 clinical trials of the rotavirus vaccine constitute blatant violations of the medical code of ethics.[109]

- ... the manufacturers' package inserts and FDA licensing documents indicate that none of the US routine childhood vaccines has been tested against a true placebo.[110]

- The entire vaccine program is based on a deliberate cover-up of true vaccine adverse event rates. This seemingly mighty fortress, carefully constructed over many decades and fortified by countless officials, researchers, and physicians - actually stands on nothing but turtles all the way down.[111]

- "In stark contrast to the (apparently unofficial) message of the medical establishment that the current vaccine schedule has been thoroughly investigated and reviewed and was found to be the best available, the schedule as a whole has NEVER been properly studied for safety or efficacy."[112]

- "Findings such as these would imply that vaccines are the main culprit behind the astronomical rise in chronic health conditions in children of the developed world and would likely cause a social and political upheaval of unprecedented proportions, both in the United States and around the globe." [113]

The Real Anthony Fauci – Robert F. Kennedy, Jr [114]

- The CDC has a $11.5 billion budget, and $4.9 billion of it is for buying, selling, and distributing vaccines. The CDC is a vaccine company.

- The CDC owns 57 vaccine patents. It can make money on the sale of every vaccine.

- The FDA gets 50% of its budget from vaccine companies.
- The NIH owns 100s of vaccine patents.
- The NIH owns half the patent for the Moderna Vaccine.
- There are five scientists who work for the NIH who worked on the vaccines and are allowed to collect $150,000 in royalties every year the vaccine is sold.
- These vaccine regulatory agencies are actually vaccine companies.
- Dr Willian Thompson, the head safety scientist for vaccine studies at the CDC for 18 years, came forward in 2019 and admitted that they were ordered to fake all the safety studies on Autism.
- Dr. William Thompson, who is currently at the CDC as of 2023, still wants the press to cover this story about the corruption at the CDC. The media will not do one interview to bring light to his story.
- 54% of Americans have a chronic disease. Vaccines are never tested on people with chronic diseases.
- Vaccine safety is ALWAYS tested in comparison to other vaccines. A vaccine safety test has NEVER been tested against a harmless placebo-like saline. In the history of any other drug safety testing, this is unheard of because it virtually renders the test useless. In other words, the ONLY thing the safety test shows is that it is as safe or safer than a previous vaccine. For example, if a new vaccine is given to a group of people and then compared to a placebo group of people who are given the meningitis vaccine, which has extreme side effects, including death, then the new vaccine may appear just as safe. It would be rendered "safe" when,

in fact, it isn't safe at all! Let's just say previous vaccines were unsafe. Then, ALL new vaccines have the bar set so high as far as safety that there is essentially no safety test at all. It is just smoke and mirrors. It looks like it's there, but it's not. Vaccine safety tests get a free pass because all the regulatory agencies benefit financially from the approval, sale, and distribution of vaccines.

- Cochrane, the highest authority on vaccine safety, and the British Medical Journal have done three giant, separate studies in 2010, 2014, and 2017 on all the literature that exists in Pub Med (127 studies) on the flu vaccine in 2010, 2014, and 2017. They determined an individual would need to get 100 vaccines to prevent ONE CASE of the flu!
- There is zero evidence that the flu vaccine prevents any hospitalization or deaths.
- The flu vaccine transmits the flu.
- Life expectancy has gone down dramatically since flu shots have been given regularly.
- There is no doctor, scientist, or vaccine expert who is willing to debate vaccine safety.[114]

CHAPTER 42

What Is the "Secret" Revealed in Plain Sight?

❧

Nature has supplied us with balance and harmony from the smallest particle within us to the infinite cosmos. There is a hidden wealth of knowledge available to you. It hides in plain sight to experience, read, and understand. The truth is also hidden within your own common sense and wisdom.

Germs are not meant to attack and destroy us, my friend. It is the opposite. You will produce germs, including viruses when you need them to help your body stay in balance. If you stay positive and let go of fears and resentment, your body and world will be filled with harmony!

Stress, in its many toxic forms, is the root cause of disease. You are your own best doctor! Look within. As Jesus once said, "The Kingdom of Heaven is within you." Don't make a Hades where your Soul resides. We need only to let go of old beliefs and practices that don't serve this truth.

You are made of star light. It is time we all shine...

The Five Biological Laws of Nature – 5BN

❧

Because German New Medicine (GNM) is Biological Medicine, what we think of as disease or cancer is called a Significant Biological Special Program (SBP).[115]

Dr Hamer discovered 5 Biological Laws that explain how our brain mediates between our psyche and our organs.

He discovered that disease is a tissue manifestation or a tissue "response" that comes from specific biological programs that get triggered in a world of many situations perceived as threats to our survival and happiness. The brain triggers our organs to *adapt* to the life shock we experience.

His scientific chart states: "Without panicking, a GNM therapist should be consulted to discuss the details [of your symptoms and disease]. We can be assured: 98% of patients survive without panic. There is no reason to be afraid!"[116]

THERE IS NO REASON TO BE AFRAID!!

In the Spanish Community, German New Medicine is called "La Medicina Sagrada" (Sacred Medicine).

Dr Hamer's Five Biological Laws:[117]

First Biological Law of Nature

Every disease originates from a serious life trauma or shock that is unexpected, sudden, intense, and isolating. This life trauma or shock was originally called "The Iron Rule of Cancer," which had three criteria.

First criterion: **The life mental shock.** Every Significant Biological Special Program (SBP) originates from a *serious, highly acute, dramatic, and isolating conflict shock* that occurs simultaneously on three levels: psyche, brain, and organ. In GNM, it is called a "DHS" (Dirk Hamer Syndrome), which is the label Dr. Hamer gave it in honor of Dirk, his son, after his tragic death.

Second criterion: **Target rings on the brain (and the organ)!** The DHS determines the location of the SBP in the brain. Picture in your mind when a pebble drops in water. We know what organ is affected because we see concentric rings on a brain CT in the exact location (brain relay) that controls the organ affected. These are sometimes referred to as lesions or edemas. In GNM, these rings are called Hamer Focus (HH). The organ affected has a *tissue response* that we call "disease." In the bigger picture, it's an *adaptation* to survive!

The third criterion is **the Psyche–Brain–Organ connection**; the course of the SBP runs simultaneously on all three levels: psyche–brain–organ. It starts with the DHS (the conflict shock) and is followed immediately by the Conflict Active (CA) phase, where the body is "buzzy and cold." Once the brain relaxes, realizes what triggered the mental shock, and comes to terms with the event, we have a ***resolution of the conflict*** (Conflictolysis – CL). This can happen after a day, a week, a month, and sometimes years! When the Post Conflict Phase (PCL) starts, we start healing! A peak will occur in the middle of the healing phase called an epic crisis (EC). After the EC, it is smooth sailing, and a normal level returns (normatonia). More explanation of this can be found in the Second Law (see graph).

Second Biological Law of Nature

The complete process from disease to resolution goes through clearly identifiable phases, two phases, to be precise — from conflict shock to its resolution and restoration of health. Psyche, brain, and body all go through the stages of this process at the *same* time.

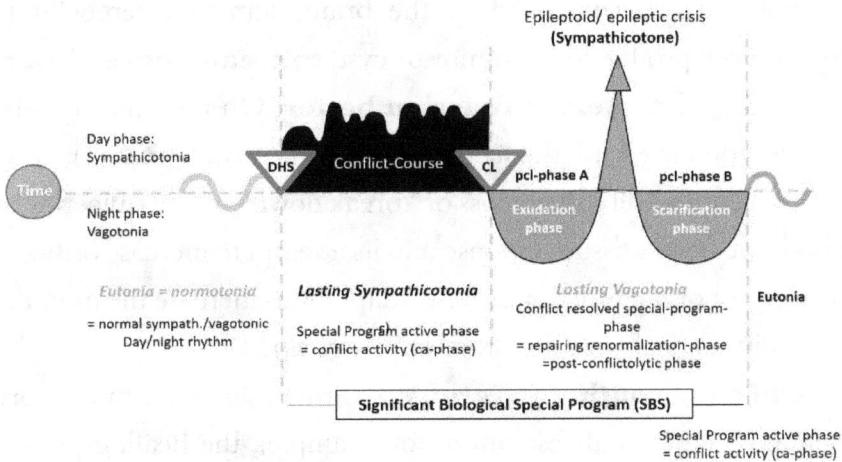

Epileptoid/ epileptic crisis
(Sympathicotone)

Day phase:
Sympathicotonia

DHS   Conflict-Course   CL   pcl-phase A   pcl-phase B

Time

Night phase:
Vagotonia

Exudation phase   Scarification phase

Eutonia = normotonia   Lasting Sympathicotonia   Lasting Vagotonia   Eutonia

= normal sympath./vagotonic   Special Program active phase   Conflict resolved special-program-phase
Day/night rhythm   = conflict activity (ca-phase)   = repairing renormalization-phase
=post-conflictolytic phase

Significant Biological Special Program (SBS)

Special Program active phase
= conflict activity (ca-phase)

CONFLICT ACTIVE PHASE: The phase following the initial shock (DHS). All activity in the body shifts to managing the conflict. The psyche is on high alert, and we experience distress and worry. Buzzy and cold!

The brain lesion (HH) corresponds to the area best suited to resolve the conflict. Its size will reflect the **intensity** of the shock or the **duration** of the conflict phase — the more significant the shock and the longer our brain is in distress about it, the larger the lesion (HH) in the brain will be.

Physically, we feel **cold, lack appetite, and cannot sleep at night**. We can lose weight, our heart can race, our blood pressure goes up, our blood sugar goes down, and we may feel nausea and dizziness. We are on high alert. This, biologically, allows us to focus and resolve the problem. The lack of sleep gives us more waking hours to find a resolution.

Organs or tissues will respond with cell growth or cell loss, depending on where in the brain the lesion (HH) occurs. For example, organs controlled by the brain stem and cerebellum increase cell production (a tumor or cyst) **to create more of the same organ to help it function better**. On the other hand, organs connected to the cerebral medulla (white matter) and cerebral cortex will suffer a loss or "break down" of cells (ulcerate). This is the body's tissue response and its attempt to increase orifices or to adjust organ function. These adaptations increase the organ's capability to deal with the situation *biologically*.

Once the conflict is resolved (through life adjustments or mental or emotional resolution, for example), the healing phase begins, and the psyche, brain, and organs heal all at the same time. This is when we go back to the ***moment*** the initial shock occurred, and we "come to terms" with it and recognize what initiated the shock, the trauma, the brain "jostle!" This is when the brain and psyche will start to relax. We recommend working with a qualified GNM Consultant because there are some individuals who are vulnerable to unforeseen reactions. (Extreme symptoms, seizures, heart attacks, and/or drastic life decisions.)

We know the conflict is resolved when we feel relief and we stop worrying about it.

Let's review... First, we have the life trauma or shock (DHS), then the Conflict Active phase. The symptoms in the Conflict Active phase are often − feeling cold, lacking an appetite, and insomnia. Possible weight loss, high blood pressure, low blood sugar. Possible nausea and dizziness. We are on high alert to focus and resolve the issue.

Once the conflict is resolved, we go into the healing stage.

HEALING STAGES: During the first stage of healing, we feel relaxed and tired to the point, quite often, of exhaustion and weakness. But our appetite is good, and our body is once again warm, perhaps even feverish for a while. This biological healing response is very adequate to what the body wants to do − restore tissue and organ functions by focusing everything on healing. Doing so causes us to stay put by making us *slightly* weak and drowsy.

The brain lesion (HH) **begins to heal** as soon as we resolve the conflict in our minds. Healing follows two phases both in brain and body. During the first phase of the healing process, an edema is formed over the lesion to protect it while it is being repaired. If big enough, it can cause some pain (headache), dizziness, vision problems, or other symptoms, depending on which brain relays are pressed by the edema. The healing of the lesion (HH) at this point can be seen on a brain scan as a bullseye, but this time, it appears blurry. Some GNM professionals say the bullseye looks like it has "bicycle spokes" or "porcupine spines."

This stage of the healing culminates with the Epileptoid Crisis (or "Epi-Crisis" or "EC" for short) — It's generally a brief healing crisis during which we experience a sharp but short relapse into the conflict phase. We may briefly feel stress symptoms, shivers, and nausea. The purpose of this short crisis is to help press and push the brain edema (HH) out because it will no longer be needed after healing has concluded. This often happens in the middle of the night while we are completely asleep.

However, let us emphasize here and add that in some extreme cases, depending on which area of the brain was affected and the organs it controls, the healing crisis ("Epi-Crisis/EC") can cause **heart attacks, strokes, asthma attacks, migraine attacks, or epileptic seizures.**

The second phase of healing begins after the "Epi-Crisis/EC," which is when the brain edema is pressed out. The lesion (HH) is now completely healed by neuroglia, which is harmless brain connective tissue. Neuroglia, or Glial Cells, are specifically useful for healing the brain. Conventional Medicine does not recognize this simple observation. Sometimes, a large accumulation of such neuroglia can be mistaken for a brain tumor, especially when we are dealing with the results of a very intense shock or one of long duration.

Organs go through the two stages of healing as well, at the same time as the brain heals. Typically, tumors that grew during the conflict phase are now broken down and re-absorbed or expelled from the body. Specialized fungi and mycobacteria are instrumental in this process. If they are not available, the tumor stays in place and encapsulates without growing any further.

Organs that lost cells during the conflict phase now regrow tissue through the creation of new cells. Sometimes, we see a sudden cell growth that is wrongly confused with a cancerous cell growth. This process of cell replenishment is aided by specialized bacteria and microbes, which make it proceed faster and better (it can also happen without them)!

Most of the symptoms we typically associate with disease can actually be an indication of healing. For example, our body repairs tissue through swelling, inflammation, infections, fever, and pain. It's very familiar to us when we observe the healing of a bee sting or a fall and scrape on the knee.

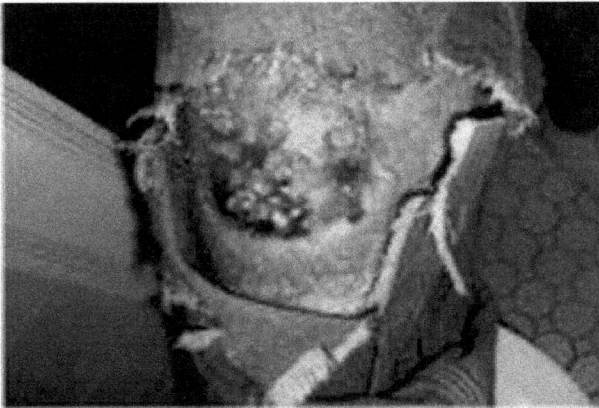

www.learninggnm.com

Many of these symptoms (pus, inflammation, swelling, pain) occur when any wound is healing. The healing of cancer is *exactly the same*. The most important point to be made here!

The intensity and length of the healing phase depend on the magnitude of the initial conflict. Because the intensity of the healing process can also cause us pain and distress, it can make healing drag on longer. Often, people are frightened by the symptoms of healing, mistaking them for disease. Pain and fear can make it hard to relax and to let the body heal.

Relapses and chronic conditions are a dragging on of the healing process. This happens when there are triggers in our environment called "TRACKS." These tracks remind us of the initial shock and set us repeatedly into conflict mode (re-experiencing the life shock), causing us to cycle again and again through conflict and healing. This is typical, for example, with allergies, arthritis, osteoarthritis, or MS, to name a few.

Here is how it happens: When we experience an intense shock, our whole system goes on high alert, and our mind sees and makes a note of all the greater details in our environment — sound, smell, and visual items are all registered subconsciously and kept in memory. The biological purpose for this is to recognize and categorize these as "possible signs of danger." When we next encounter them, our system will react by sending a signal of danger to our brain. This evokes the memory of the past trauma and its respective protective response. These are called "TRACKS" in GNM. Conventional medicine would call these *allergies*.

Our memory will let go of these memories or "imprints" once we are healed. But sometimes, some memories linger longer, causing us to relapse. These relapses are very short, the conflict phase being imperceptible, but the healing phase is what we notice — swelling, runny nose, rashes, etc. Our body responds to the trigger for protection to prevent a new conflict like the one we experienced the last time. This is what we normally call an *allergy*.

Biological purpose. Once the healing is complete, normal functioning comes back, and more importantly, all affected organs are *fortified* to prevent future issues with what is now perceived as a vulnerable part of our system. If a future shock of a similar nature were to occur, this body part would be stronger and better equipped to deal with it. One of the best observations of this is when we break a bone. Once a fracture is healed, there is an overproduction of bone calcium on the healed break.

Let us tell you the story of......
"DUST ALLERGIES" by **Klaus-Dieter D., Germany**[118]

October 26, 2008
40 years of Dust Allergies gone?

"I have had a terrible dust allergy for over 40 years. At least, I thought I did because I always had to be careful about keeping the house clean and, above all, dust-free.

Whenever there was even the slightest evidence of dust or the finest traces of any powder in a room, I had to sneeze continually for about three hours and was constantly sniffing because my nose was always running.

After having become familiar with GNM, I started asking myself why it was that I constantly had to sneeze and sniffle when this all started and what the "track" (trigger) was that kept activating the condition (the "allergy").

After recently moving into a new house that wasn't quite finished yet, my allergy really took off, which indicated that I had set on a track! So, I continued thinking hard about what the reason could possibly be.

I was rewarded with a sudden memory of having been hit by rocks three times in the head while playing with my buddies in the ruins of Berlin. It was the only playing area the children of that city had available in 1955. It was, of course, terribly dusty there because the walls of ruined houses were still collapsing, and clouds of dust would explode. In all that dirt, I was accidentally hit three times in the head by a rock. I had to go to the doctor, and each time, a concussion was diagnosed.

The moment I remembered these events, the sneezing and my runny nose stopped - and they have done so right up to this moment! In the meantime, I have even been in a terribly dusty garage. There, a marble polisher had been cutting up his marble slabs for 30 years but had never once cleaned the garage. I swept out all that dust with a broom, and the dust clouds just flew. I was literally working in a fog of dust! However, I didn't have to sneeze or sniffle even once - neither during the rest of the building period, nor afterward, nor during all the weeks after that."

Klaus-Dieter D.

GNM Explanation: The biological conflict (DHS) linked to the nasal membrane is a "stink conflict" ("This situation stinks!") or a "scent conflict" in the sense of not being able to "scent" - sniff out – an immediate danger or threat; in the case at hand: the rocks flying towards the head. – During the conflict-active phase, the nasal membrane ulcerates, causing tissue loss to widen the nasal passage so that the danger can be better identified (sniffed out). During the healing phase, the ulcerated area is replenished, accompanied by swelling, causing a stuffed-up nose; other typical healing symptoms are a runny nose, nasal discharge, and sneezing to get rid of remnants of the repair process (symptoms of a common cold). When a DHS occurs, the mind picks up all the components that are considered important in association with the conflict. In this case, **dust was established as a track**. The biological significance of tracks is to serve as a warning signal, saying, "Watch out! Last time you were around dust you were in danger!" Thus, whenever the brain registers "dust," the conflict-related Significant Biological Special Program (SBP) is quickly re-activated with instant sneezing and a runny nose. What is commonly referred to as an "allergy" or an "allergic reaction" are the track(s) that were established at the moment of the conflict shock. The first step to breaking the track cycle is to identify the original conflict. With the awareness that DUST does no longer pose a danger (for our friend, the dust in the ruins in Berlin is, in the present time, no longer a concern), the psyche can now delete "dust" (the "warning") from its memory, and the "allergy" is instantly gone – and this after 40 years!

NOTE: The diagnosis of a "dust allergy" can cause a new "dust track," causing, for those that don't understand, a chronic allergic condition. With the knowledge of GNM, a person suffering from "allergies" is in a position to complete the healing once and for all. (From www.learninggnm.com) [119]

Third Biological Law of Nature

All SBPs are directly related to the embryology of the human cell layers: Endoderm, Mesoderm, and Ectoderm. These are called "Germ Layers," not to be confused with germs as microbes.

In other words, the psyche, brain, and organs are biologically connected, and this is once again observed in the stages of evolutionary and embryonic development of the human being.

Okay, stay with us here. We have the older part of our brain, called the endoderm and old Mesoderm. In most texts of German New Medicine, these tissues are colored yellow and orange. The new part of the brain is the new Mesoderm and ectoderm. The new Mesoderm, in GNM diagrams, is colored dark orange, and the ectoderm is colored red.

Remember, the original definition of germ is "To grow outward, to sprout." The endoderm is associated with the food we eat and the alimentary process. It's associated with the path our food travels through the body, everything from our lips, mouth, esophagus, stomach, small intestines, liver, gall bladder, large intestines, and out. The Brain Stem controls all those organs.

In GNM, we *further divide the Mesoderm into two parts*. The Old Mesoderm and the New Mesoderm. The Old Mesoderm is associated with corium skin (under the skin, our original protective skin), sweat glands, breast glands, and more. The Old Mesoderm is controlled by the Cerebellum.

The New Mesoderm is associated with the bones, bone marrow, blood cells, tooth dentin, heart muscles and valves, blood vessels, lymph nodes, spleen, and more. The Cerebral Medulla controls all of those. Finally, we have the Ectoderm, which is associated with the Outer Skin! Are you seeing the puzzle pieces coming together!?! Isn't that amazing? We hope you are in awe of whoever you consider your creator!

In most texts of German New Medicine, these tissues are colored yellow, orange, dark orange, and red. We have the older part of our brain called the Endoderm and Old Mesoderm. The new part of the brain is the New Mesoderm and Ectoderm.

It has been observed in a woman's womb that the human organism develops by passing through all the typical phases that it went through during its evolution as a species. As we follow the growth of the human embryo, it is as if we are observing an accelerated version of the evolution of man. We see the appearance, one after the other, of the three main germ layers. From these layers, our organs grow, corresponding to each layer.

From here, it is easy to follow the connections between brain areas and organs, as well as the purpose of each organ — and the biological purpose each organ serves at the time of its appearance and full development.

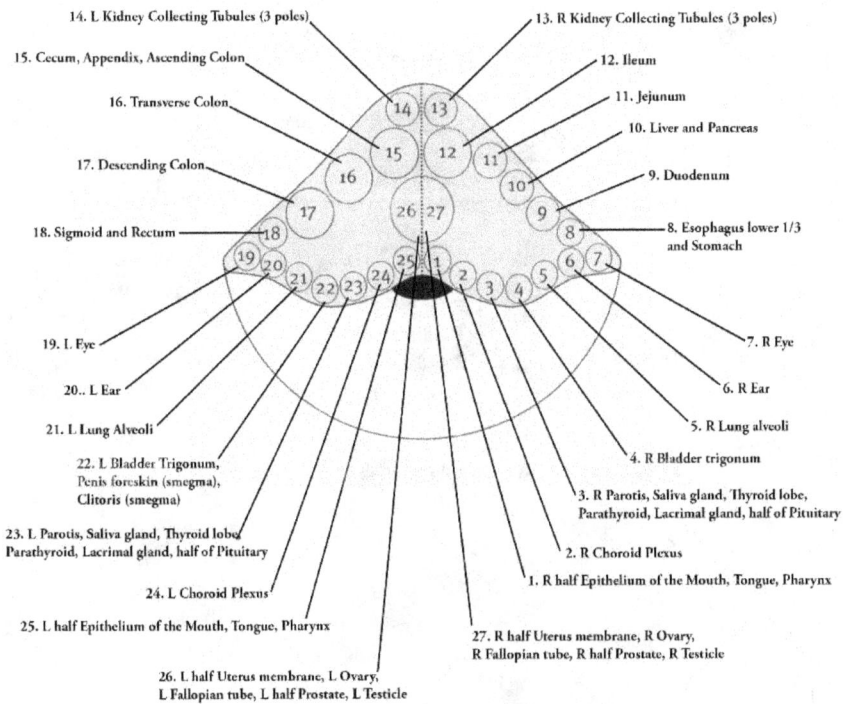

14. L Kidney Collecting Tubules (3 poles)

15. Cecum, Appendix, Ascending Colon

16. Transverse Colon

17. Descending Colon

18. Sigmoid and Rectum

19. L Eye

20.. L Ear

21. L Lung Alveoli

22. L Bladder Trigonum, Penis foreskin (smegma), Clitoris (smegma)

23. L Parotis, Saliva gland, Thyroid lobe Parathyroid, Lacrimal gland, half of Pituitary

24. L Choroid Plexus

25. L half Epithelium of the Mouth, Tongue, Pharynx

26. L half Uterus membrane, L Ovary, L Fallopian tube, L half Prostate, L Testicle

13. R Kidney Collecting Tubules (3 poles)

12. Ileum

11. Jejunum

10. Liver and Pancreas

9. Duodenum

8. Esophagus lower 1/3 and Stomach

7. R Eye

6. R Ear

5. R Lung alveoli

4. R Bladder trigonum

3. R Parotis, Saliva gland, Thyroid lobe, Parathyroid, Lacrimal gland, half of Pituitary

2. R Choroid Plexus

1. R half Epithelium of the Mouth, Tongue, Pharynx

27. R half Uterus membrane, R Ovary, R Fallopian tube, R half Prostate, R Testicle

www.gnminstitute.com

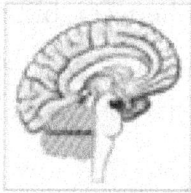

CEREBELLUM – ORGAN – RELATION

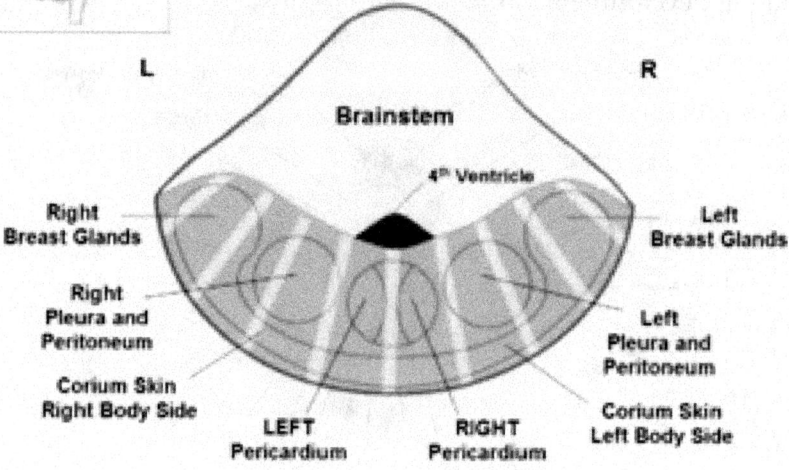

L   R

Brainstem

4th Ventricle

Right Breast Glands

Left Breast Glands

Right Pleura and Peritoneum

Left Pleura and Peritoneum

Corium Skin Right Body Side

LEFT Pericardium

RIGHT Pericardium

Corium Skin Left Body Side

© Dr. med. Mag. theol. Ryke Geerd Hamer

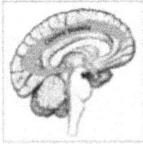

CEREBRAL MEDULLA – ORGAN – RELATION

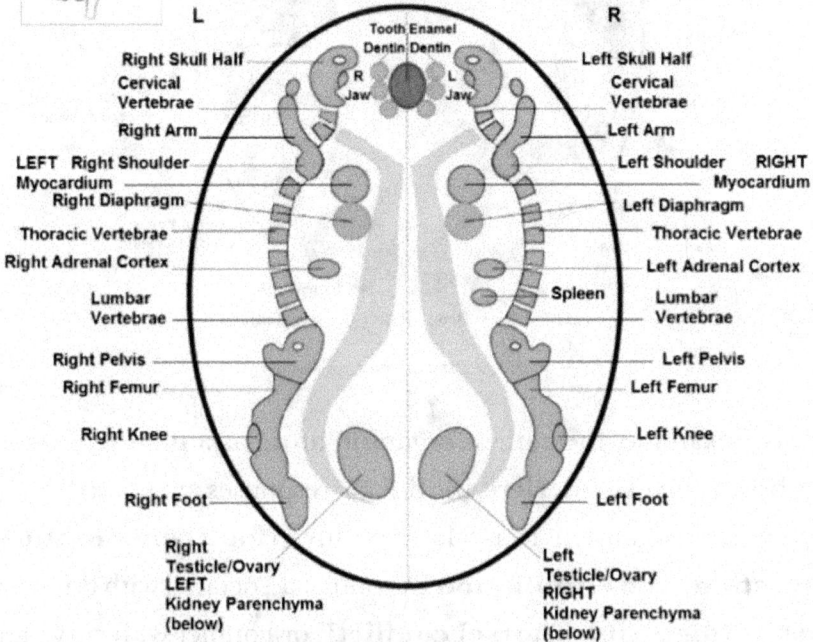

L   R

Tooth Enamel
Dentin Dentin

Right Skull Half
Cervical Vertebrae   R Jaw   L Jaw   Left Skull Half
                                                    Cervical Vertebrae
Right Arm   Left Arm

LEFT   Right Shoulder   Left Shoulder   RIGHT
Myocardium   Myocardium
        Right Diaphragm   Left Diaphragm

Thoracic Vertebrae   Thoracic Vertebrae

Right Adrenal Cortex   Left Adrenal Cortex

Lumbar Vertebrae   Spleen   Lumbar Vertebrae

Right Pelvis   Left Pelvis
Right Femur   Left Femur

Right Knee   Left Knee

Right Foot   Left Foot

Right
Testicle/Ovary   Left
LEFT   Testicle/Ovary
Kidney Parenchyma   RIGHT
(below)   Kidney Parenchyma
                                                    (below)

© Dr. med. Mag. theol. Ryke Geerd Hamer

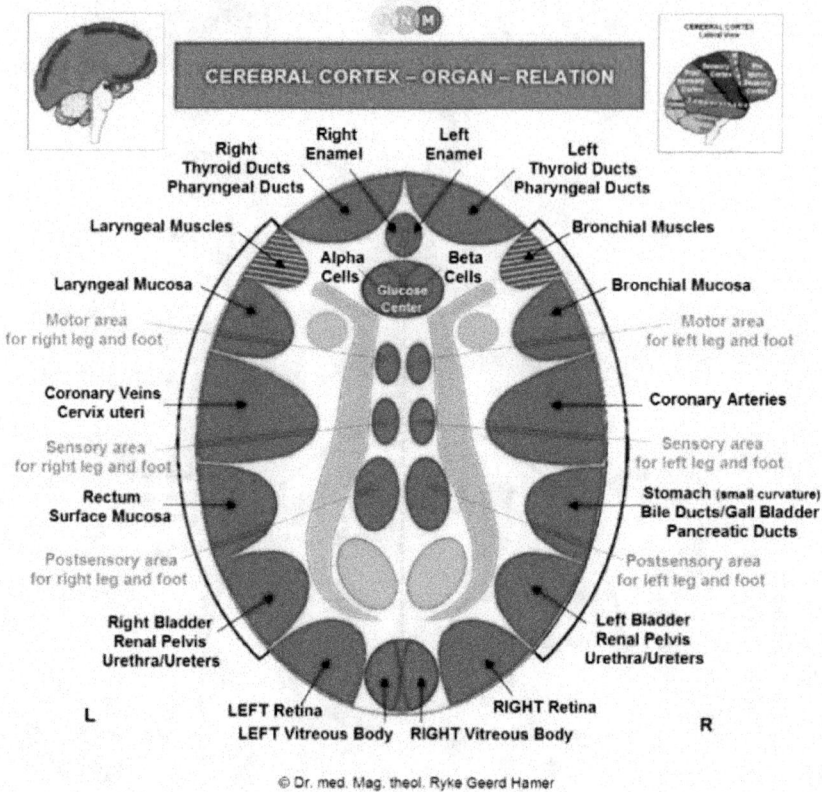

CEREBRAL CORTEX – ORGAN – RELATION

Right Enamel — Left Enamel

Right Thyroid Ducts Pharyngeal Ducts — Left Thyroid Ducts Pharyngeal Ducts

Laryngeal Muscles — Bronchial Muscles

Alpha Cells — Beta Cells

Glucose Center

Laryngeal Mucosa — Bronchial Mucosa

Motor area for right leg and foot — Motor area for left leg and foot

Coronary Veins Cervix uteri — Coronary Arteries

Sensory area for right leg and foot — Sensory area for left leg and foot

Rectum Surface Mucosa — Stomach (small curvature) Bile Ducts/Gall Bladder Pancreatic Ducts

Postsensory area for right leg and foot — Postsensory area for left leg and foot

Right Bladder Renal Pelvis Urethra/Ureters — Left Bladder Renal Pelvis Urethra/Ureters

L

LEFT Retina LEFT Vitreous Body — RIGHT Retina RIGHT Vitreous Body

R

© Dr. med. Mag. theol. Ryke Geerd Hamer

For example, the earliest organism arose at a time when only the brainstem existed. Here, the disease responses are related to *pure survival,* and organ activity is related mostly to **food consumption, digestion, and elimination**. A conflict associated with this layer is an **"indigestible morsel conflict"** or conflict with survival.

The more complex organ systems were created to reflect the higher complexity of function required, including a protective skin, a nerve-sense system, skeletal and muscle systems, the five senses, etc. These new organs correspond to the appearance of more differentiation in the brain as well, culminating with the development of the brain cortex. The brain cortex is where complex thinking processes happen, and our thoughts and ideas are registered. It's where we have a *sense of identity, territorial belonging, ownership, and more complex desires* than the single-minded urge for eating and survival.

In 1991, Dr. Hamer was presented with the brain scan of a patient and nothing else. Here is what is documented:

"After I presented a lecture in Vienna in May 1991, a doctor gave me a brain-computer tomogram (CT) of a patient. In the presence of 20 of his colleagues, among them radiologists and computer tomography experts, he asked me to tell him what symptoms the patient had and which type of conflicts *were related to them. I was asked to conclude the condition of the other two levels from the brain level. I diagnosed from the brain CT a freshly bleeding bladder carcinoma in the healing phase, an old prostate carcinoma, a diabetic condition, an old bronchial carcinoma, and a sensory paralysis of a certain area in the body - and for each of these, the corresponding conflicts that the patient must have experienced. At this point, the doctor stood up in front of all his colleagues and said, 'Dr. Hamer, congratulations! Five diagnoses - five successes! The patient had exactly what you said. And you were even able to differentiate what symptoms he had in the past and which symptom he has right now.'"*

Fourth Biological Law of Nature

There is a correlation between the brain, the germ layers (cell layers), and microbes. Germs like mycobacteria, fungi, bacteria, and TB bacteria have a symbiotic relationship with our cells. Germs break down and degrade overgrowths or help build back cells during any cancer or disease process.

In other words, bacteria, fungi, and viruses are intimately involved in the healing processes in the body. The choice of which microbial form should be used by

the body depends on the tissue affected and the respective part of the brain it relates to.

We all *now know* that germs, bacteria, and fungi are not the bad guys!! We eat yogurt, we drink kombucha, and we eat all kinds of fermented foods because germs are here to keep *creating harmony*. Germs evolved parallel to our own evolution, and they were (and still are) part of our internal ecosystem, in charge of *always* maintaining balance. Each organ system has specific microbes that, when necessary, will help keep those organs healthy.

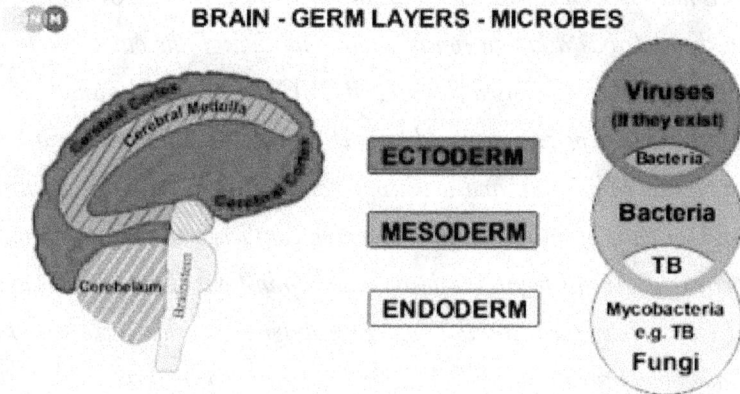

BRAIN - GERM LAYERS - MICROBES

Cerebral Cortex
Cerebral Medulla
Cerebral Cortex
Cerebellum
Brainstem

ECTODERM

MESODERM

ENDODERM

Viruses
(if they exist)
Bacteria

Bacteria

TB

Mycobacteria
e.g. TB

Fungi

www.learninggnm.com

In the case of a "death fright conflict" (GNM term), such as a cancer diagnosis or a threat of war that has passed, like WWII, the brain activates Tuberculin Bacteria (TB) to break down the extra lung cells that have grown to "help" breathe and better to cope with the shock. The active TB bacteria will be interpreted as tuberculosis; the extra lung cells will be erroneously labeled as lung cancer.

During the healing phase of a death fright, patients will often have bloody sputum, coughing, fatigue, fever, inflammation, and pain. If antibiotics are used, as was the case in millions of people recovering from the shock of WWII, the cells will remain in place and encapsulate, forming what looks like a lung tumor on an X-ray. Although these are harmless, they may be found on an X-ray years later and create a new conflict that GNM would call a "death fright conflict," especially if a doctor diagnoses the person with "lung cancer." If the person is not aware of GNM, they will trigger their brain to relapse into another death shock.

Germs only get activated during the healing phase. As soon as the conflict is resolved and healing begins, a signal is sent to activate the bacteria or fungi needed for that specific function. The rest of the time – when we are healthy or when we are in conflict mode, they simply and harmlessly exist in smaller quantities in the body. Remember, we have four times more bacteria than cells. Active or not, the role of bacteria, fungi, and viruses is always to optimize healing. They are otherwise always harmless. To reiterate: Germs are NOT THE BAD GUYS!

Conventional/Contemporary medical science does not accept or desire to address the monumental findings of Dr. Hamer in this and many other areas outlined in German New Medicine. For that reason, they do not even follow the stages of disease and healing. They do not understand the processes typical of those stages, and – logically, they do not grasp the role of microbes in our body. In fact, they make theoretical speculations that have no basis in the scientific method. Conventional medicine is *only* interested in drug or surgical procedures, and those only *alleviate* symptoms. Many diseases are highly misunderstood!

A doctor will identify the existence of bacteria once it appears in the second phase of healing as a ***disease process***. The typical swelling, discharges, fevers, and other symptoms that appear with the activity of bacteria are labeled a disease. Medication is used to destroy the microbes, and that *(unfortunately) suppresses a perfectly natural healing process*. This not only causes a slowing down of healing but also introduces new harm in the form of medication toxicity and the destruction of much-needed bacteria.

So, what are the germs useful for? With the help of bacteria, fungi, and viruses, our body breaks down cysts and tumors, liquefies, and further decomposes dead tissue and cells, and turns them into a form easy to eliminate. This happens through the usual pathways — skin, liver, kidneys, colon, and lungs. Without these pathways, our body would become septic, waste matter would not be dealt with properly, and the inner balance of our body would be upset.

"In certain tissues, microbes will be used to repair the damaged cells by building back areas of tissue loss. In ectodermal organs, bacteria help to restore the cell loss. Streptococcus bacteria, for instance, assist healing in the throat (strep throat), pneumococcus bacteria restore the bronchial mucosa, gonococcus bacteria work in the urogenital area, and the Helicobacter pylori repairs the stomach and pylorus lining. This, however, only happens when the ulceration in the conflict-active phase reaches far into the tissue. Otherwise, the healing process takes place without microbes." (www.learninggnm.com)[120]

Let's look at a case study of the typical sore throat and cough from GNM perspective.

Case study on April 2010

CLIENT: 20-year-old left-handed female

Subjective Complaint: Sore throat, cough for a few days, and a fever. She indicates that the symptoms began four days ago on a Friday. She reports that it began as a sore throat and later progressed to a cough with a fever and generalized fatigue.

Observation: The client presented with a slight fever, fatigue, and constant cough. Organs affected: Bronchial mucosa and upper 2/3 of esophagus.

Embryonic Germ layer: ectoderm Brain Control center: cerebral cortex (sensory cortex) GNM

Explanation: Constant cough is related to a scare-fright conflict. During the healing phase, the ulcerated bronchial lining is replenished, typically accompanied by coughing, fatigue, and fever. A sore throat is related to the conflict of not wanting to swallow/accept "a morsel" (situation or an event). During the healing phase, the ulceration of the upper part of the esophagus is replenished, which causes a sore throat and swelling.

GNM Understanding: After discussing the conflicts involved, the client mentioned that she was working on a school portfolio project, which was due last Friday. She indicated that on Tuesday of the same week, she was working on her portfolio when her computer crashed, and she thought she lost all of her work (her DHS). She states that she became concerned that she might not be able to turn in the work on time. However, a couple of days later, she was able to recover her work and courier the portfolio in time. It was on Friday, after the conflict was resolved, that her symptoms first appeared. Results: The client was able to make the connection with the GNM explanation that she was actually already in the healing phase of a Biological Special Program (SBP) that was triggered by the unexpected shock of fearing she would lose her work and that it would not be handed in on time (which was "hard to swallow"). (www.learninggnm.com) [121]

Fifth Biological Law of Nature: The "Quintessence"

Every so-called "disease" is part of a significant biological special program (SBP) of nature, comprehensible in the context of our evolution.

The fifth biological natural law is the Quintessence of German New Medicine. It indicates that nothing in nature is meaningless or "malignant," as we have been taught. For each disease, DHS that catches an individual "on the wrong foot" triggers a Significant Biological Special Program (SBP), which assists the organism in resolving the actual conflict situation. Even the "constellations" (two SBPs in opposite positions in the brain) can now be understood as meaningful, temporary meta-programs. [93]

In other words, disease is a meaningful process and not an accident.

Once we realize the implications of Dr. Hamer's findings, we can reach the conclusion that nothing in nature is random and all processes have a purpose, including those occurring in our own bodies.

Based on the solid research behind such conclusions, we can now take a second look at what ails us, and we are better equipped to find the cause and the meaning of each biological process. More importantly, we can connect physical symptoms to deeper and more significant themes related to our own nature, life purpose, and character.

Life-threatening diseases such as cancer, heart disease, and autoimmune diseases can now be understood and addressed in a way that can lead to health and not to death, as we have been taught to believe.

We now see that our diseases reflect our life challenges and that our body is well equipped to lead us safely to the other side, back to health. Of course, with the new understanding of this beautiful biological process, we also learn ways to help ourselves through it. We can now let go of harmful interventions and medications, and instead, we can take all the adequate measures that support our body rather than handicap it.

Armed with new knowledge, we can avoid harmful diagnosis shocks by reaching for a better explanation of what is happening to our body — then, we can form conclusions based on solid biological laws and on a commonsense view that is based on true observation. These observations and proof come from more than tens of thousands of GNM cases.

German New Medicine consists of educating the patient by explaining what is happening and ***taking away the fear***. Once the process is understood, the nature of the conflict must be found. If it's not yet resolved, counseling and discussion aim to lead to a resolution of the disease-inducing shock and conflict.

Instead of focusing on the symptoms alone and then targeting them with conventional drugs, surgery, or even holistic treatments aiming at getting rid of them, German New Medicine follows the natural progression of the disease. GNM takes measures to resolve existing stress while assisting the body in its healing. Special care is taken during the healing phase to avoid complications through either relapse into conflict or through too intense and harmful healing symptoms.

Our spiritual growth is part of all healing, and as such, the themes uncovered by German New Medicine can enhance our journey and bring clarity into who we are and how to improve ourselves. With more trust in our body and inner knowing, we can embark with more assurance on a journey of enlightenment. Knowing that our body is always taking care of our survival and needs, we can embrace it as our partner in life and not an enemy that needs to be constantly feared, watched, and controlled.

"All so-called diseases have a special biological meaning. While we used to regard Mother Nature as fallible and had the audacity to believe that she constantly made mistakes and caused breakdowns (malignant, senseless, degenerative cancerous growths, etc.), we can now see, as the scales fall from our eyes, that it was our ignorance and pride that were and are the only foolishness in our cosmos. Blinded, we brought upon ourselves the senseless, soulless, and brutal medicine. Full of wonder, we can now understand for the first time that Nature is orderly (we already knew that), and every occurrence in Nature is meaningful, even in the framework of the whole, and that the events we call diseases are not senseless disturbances to be repaired by aspiring sorcerers. Nothing in nature is meaningless, malignant or diseased." -Dr. Med. Ryke Geerd Hamer (1935-2017) –(www.learninggnm.com)

Afterword – So, Where Do We Go From Here?

❧

This book reveals some hidden truths that will help you understand how wonderfully and divinely you are made by God. Nature has given you the gift of health and the ability to heal from disease. Disease does not come from bacteria, fungi, and viruses as Big Pharma would have us believe. Disease comes from many toxins and biological shocks we encounter daily.

To recap, the disease is a tissue manifestation or a tissue "response" that comes from specific biological programs that get triggered in a world of many situations perceived **as threats to our survival and happiness.**

These threats are called "biological shocks or conflicts" in German New Medicine. They are called stress or toxic thoughts by most of us. They are individual perceptions of our environment, and the brain and body tissue support us when we feel threatened. What we think of as germs and bacteria have evolved right along with our cells throughout our evolution *for a purpose.* The solution to our illnesses can be found in the cause.

German New Medicine – the 5 Biological Laws Dr. Hamer discovered present us with answers and solutions to cancer and disease that truly work.

There are 120 disease programs clearly explained from the root cause to the healing stages by Dr. Ryke Hamer, MD.

There are many blogs by Ilsedora Laker on her site www.gnmonlineseminars.com. She is the CEO and main presenter at the GNM Institute of German New Medicine in Toronto, Canada.

There is also a comprehensive understanding of GNM on the website www.learninggnm.com. by Caroline Markolin, Ph.D.

These are amazing resources to help you understand the FUTURE OF MEDICINE is here now!

Biographies

Dr. Robyn R. DeSautel is a dedicated healthcare professional with a wealth of experience spanning over 29 years. Her unwavering commitment to patient well-being led her to pursue a Doctor of Chiropractic degree, driven by her passion for facilitating healing without reliance on pharmaceuticals or surgical interventions. Dr. DeSautel firmly believes in empowering patients by fostering an understanding of their body's innate healing abilities, demonstrating that self-healing and the reversal of chronic conditions such as Neuropathy are indeed achievable.

In 1988, Dr. DeSautel graduated with distinction from Wartburg University in Waverly, Iowa, earning her Bachelor of Science degree. Subsequently, she excelled at the University of Western States in Portland, Oregon, graduating at the top of her class with a Doctorate Degree in chiropractic.

For over 23 years, Dr. DeSautel successfully owned and operated one of Seattle's largest and busiest multidisciplinary clinics. Having served an impressive 24,000 patients and overseeing more than 270,400 patient visits, her clinic garnered accolades for its outstanding service. Additionally, Dr. DeSautel contributed her expertise as a board member on the directors' panel of three other esteemed healthcare clinics.

David Lloyd has been an educator since 1988. He has been in Health and Wellness for over 12 years. Holding degrees in Education and Music, he works as a Certified Yoga Teacher, Reiki Master, CECP (Certified Emotion Code Practitioner) from Discover Healing and Dr. Bradley Nelson, D.C. He is also a creative writer, a poet, and a musician.

Lloyd has completed the GNM Course for Medical Professionals and the Advanced Clinician's Program through The GNM Institute in Toronto, Canada. He has self-healed more than 23 ailments in his own body by understanding the 5 Biological Laws of Nature and the discoveries of Dr. Ryke Geerd Hamer. He sends a burst of confidence *to you* so that you will also know the secrets of self-healing unearthed in this book!

End Notes

1   Turtles All The Way Down https://tinyurl.com/turtlesbookchap1eng

2   Where There Is Light by Paramahansa Yogananda pp 26 – 27

3   www.gnmonlineseminars.com Ilsedora Laker, CEO and Dean of the GNM Institute

4   *The Private Science of Louis Pasteur,* by Gerald Geisen

5   https://en.m.wikipedia.org/wiki/Flat_Earth

6   https://www.britannica.com/biography/Rudolf-Virchow

7   Image designed by Dr Marizelle Arce terraindoctor.com

8   Dr. William Trebing, Goodbye Germ Theory p 155

9   Electric Body, Electric Health by Eileen Day McKusick p 42

10 Pasteur: Plagiarist and Imposter; The Germ Theory Exploded, 1942, p 30

11 Bechamp or Pasteur? A Lost Chapter in the History of Biology, By Ethel Hume 1919
    and Pasteur: Plagiarist, Imposter; The Germ theory Exploded by R.B. Pearson 1942
    Note from the publisher of both books admin@adistantmirror.com.au 2017

12 The Truth About Contagion (Original title: The Contagion Myth) by Thomas S.
    Cowan, MD and Sally Fallon Morell

13 The Truth About Contagion by Thomas S. Cowan, MD and Sally Fallon Morell p 5

14 The Truth About Contagion by Thomas S. Cowan, MD and Sally Fallon Morell p 7

15 *The Private Science of Louis Pasteur,* by Gerald Geisen, p 151

16 Notes on Nursing, Florence Nightingale 1st ed. 1860 p.32

17 What Really Makes You Ill? Why Everything You Thought You Knew About Disease
    is Wrong by Dawn Lester and David Parker

18 The Truth About Contagion by Thomas S. Cowan, MD and Sally Fallon Morell p 3

19 The Truth About Contagion by Thomas S. Cowan, MD and Sally Fallon Morell p 4

20 The Truth About Contagion by Thomas S. Cowan, MD and Sally Fallon Morell p 4

21 Dr Stefan Lanka, Dr Andrew Kaufman, MD, Dr Thomas Cowan, MD, Dean Danes –
    Freedom Talk 5

22 The Private Science of Louis Pasteur, by Gerald Geisen, p 181

23 The Private Science of Louis Pasteur, by Gerald Geisen, p 157

24 What Really Makes You Ill: why everything you thought you knew about disease is wrong p.185-186

25 The Private Science of Louis Pasteur, by Gerald Geisen, p 241

26 The Private Science of Louis Pasteur, by Gerald Geisen, p 251

27 The Private Science of Louis Pasteur, by Gerald Geisen, p 215

28 The Private Science of Louis Pasteur, by Gerald Geisen, p 198

29 *What Really Makes You Ill: why everything you thought you knew about disease is wrong* p169-171

30 Pasteur: Plagiarist and Imposter; The Germ Theory Exploded, 1942, p 28

31 https://www.britannica.com/biography/Rudolf-Virchow

32 Bechamp or Pasteur? By Ethel Hume p 245

33 Dr. William Trebing, Goodbye Germ Theory p 151

34 2002 textbook Molecular Biology of the Cell

35 Dr. William Trebing, Goodbye Germ Theory p 155

36 1998 article titled, "Physical Properties and Heavy-metal Uptake of Encapsulated Escherichia Coli Expressing a Metal Binding Gene," from What Really Makes You Ill.

37 Dr. William Trebing, Goodbye Germ Theory p 154

38 Notes on Nursing, Florence Nightingale 1st ed. 1860 and
Pasteur: Plagiarist, Imposter The Germ Theory Exploded by R. B. Pearson p 13

39 Dr. William Trebing, Goodbye Germ Theory p 155

40 Co-Senior Investigator, Ken Caldwell, PhD

41 The End of Covid, The Narrative (Act 2), Video 11, The "Proof" of Contagion: Dawn Lester, Mike Stone & Jacob Diaz

42 The End of Covid, The Narrative (Act 2), Video 11, The "Proof" of Contagion: Dawn Lester, Mike Stone & Jacob Diaz

43 The Expectation Effect by David Robson p 2 – 3

44 The Expectation Effect by David Robson p 7

45 "Diseases, Memories of Evolution" by Dr. Robert Guinée; based on the work of Doctor R.G. Hamer (French title: Maladies, mémoires de l'évolution / Dr Robert Guinée ; basé sur les travaux du Docteur R.G. Hamer)

46 https://www.gnmonlineseminars.com/treatment-in-the-gnm/

47 www.learninggnm.com

48 www.learninggnm.com

49 1921 by the Hygienic Laboratory #123 https://www.scribd.com/document/578758384/20210424-Spanische-Grippe-Studie

50 www.learninggnm.com

51 https://www.sott.net/article/340948-Biologist-wins-Supreme-Court-case-proving-that-the-measles-virus-does-not-exist

52 Ekaterina Sugak, Naturopath www.ekaterinasugak.com

53 CPE - Control Experiment - 21 April 2021 - English version (odysee.com)

54 VIRUS MANIA: Avian Flu (H5N1), Cervical Cancer (HPV), SARS, BSE, Hepatitis

C, AIDS, Polio...How the Medical Industry Continually Invents Epidemics, Making Billion-Dollar Profits at Our Expense by Torsten Engelbrecht, Dr Claus Kohnlein, Dr Samantha Bailey, MD, Dr Stefano Scoglio, MD

55   What Really Makes You Ill? Why Everything You Thought You Knew About Disease is Wrong by Dawn Lester and David Parker p 89

56   Confessions of a Medical Heretic by Dr. Robert Mendelsohn, MD

57   Symbiotic Planet by Dr Margulis

58   Goodbye Germ Theory by Dr William Trebing p 155

59   What Really Makes You Ill? Why Everything You Thought You Knew About Disease is Wrong by Dawn Lester and David Parker p 53

60   What Really Makes You Ill? Why Everything You Thought You Knew About Disease is Wrong by Dawn Lester and David Parker p 54

61   1948 John Paul of Yale University, International Poliomyelitis Congress

62   1941 Scientific Journal ARCHIVES of Pediatrics

63   May 1955 Carl Eklund

64   Fear of the Invisible: A Hidden Epidemic by Janine Roberts p 66

65   Fear of the Invisible: A Hidden Epidemic by Janine Roberts p 66

66   Vaccination, Greg Beattie p 53

67   Virus Mania, Good-bye Germ Theory, What Really makes you sick

68   What Really Makes You Ill? Why Everything You Thought You Knew About Disease is Wrong by Dawn Lester and David Parker p 54

69   Invisible Rainbow by Arthur Firstenberg p 107 – 109

70   Vaccine Whistleblower: Exposing Autism Research Fraud at the CDC by Kevin Barry

71   VIRUS MANIA: Avian Flu (H5N1), Cervical Cancer (HPV), SARS, BSE, Hepatitis C, AIDS, Polio...How the Medical Industry Continually Invents Epidemics, Making Billion-Dollar Profits at Our Expense by Torsten Engelbrecht, Dr Claus Kohnlein, Dr Samantha Bailey, MD, Dr Stefano Scoglio, MD pp 90-152

72   Dr. Heinz Ludwig Sanger, Emeritus Professor of Molecular Biology and Virology, Max-Planck-Institute for Biochemistry, Munich

73   Vaccination - Genocide in the third Millennium? By Stefan Lanka and Karl Krafeld read more at: https://www.preciousorganics.com.au/pages/dr-stefan-lanka-exposes-the-viral-fraud

74   http://www.virusmyth.com/aids/controversy.htm

75   Reinharth Kurth, director of the Robert Koch Institute in Der Speigel, September 9th, 2004

76   Goodbye Germ Theory by Dr William Trebing p 159

77   Dr. Stefan Lanka: "All claims about viruses as pathogens are false" report.

78   Goodbye Germ Theory by Dr William Trebing p 159

79   VIRUS MANIA: Avian Flu (H5N1), Cervical Cancer (HPV), SARS, BSE, Hepatitis C, AIDS, Polio...How the Medical Industry Continually Invents Epidemics, Making

Billion-Dollar Profits at Our Expense by Torsten Engelbrecht, Dr Claus Kohnlein, Dr Samantha Bailey, MD, Dr Stefano Scoglio, MD p 161-164

80 "The Real Anthony Fauci" Bill Gates, Big Pharma, and the Global War on Democracy and Public Health - by Robert F. Kennedy, Jr.

81 www.Learninggnm.com

82 VIRUS MANIA: Avian Flu (H5N1), Cervical Cancer (HPV), SARS, BSE, Hepatitis C, AIDS, Polio…How the Medical Industry Continually Invents Epidemics, Making Billion-Dollar Profits at Our Expense by Torsten Engelbrecht, Dr Claus Kohnlein, Dr Samantha Bailey, MD, Dr Stefano Scoglio, MD p 116

83 Haverkos, Harry, Disease Manifestation among Homosexual Men with Acquired Immunodeficiency Syndrome: A Possible Role of Nitrites in Kaposi's Sarcoma, Sexually Transmitted Diseases, October- December 1985, pp. 203-208

84 Krieger, Terry; Caceres, Cesar; The Unnoticed Link in AIDS cases, Wall Street Journal, 24 October 1985

85 VIRUS MANIA: Avian Flu (H5N1), Cervical Cancer (HPV), SARS, BSE, Hepatitis C, AIDS, Polio…How the Medical Industry Continually Invents Epidemics, Making Billion-Dollar Profits at Our Expense by Torsten Engelbrecht, Dr Claus Kohnlein, Dr Samantha Bailey, MD, Dr Stefano Scoglio, MD p 103

86 VIRUS MANIA: Avian Flu (H5N1), Cervical Cancer (HPV), SARS, BSE, Hepatitis C, AIDS, Polio…How the Medical Industry Continually Invents Epidemics, Making Billion-Dollar Profits at Our Expense by Torsten Engelbrecht, Dr Claus Kohnlein, Dr Samantha Bailey, MD, Dr Stefano Scoglio, MD p 167

87 VIRUS MANIA: Avian Flu (H5N1), Cervical Cancer (HPV), SARS, BSE, Hepatitis C, AIDS, Polio…How the Medical Industry Continually Invents Epidemics, Making Billion-Dollar Profits at Our Expense by Torsten Engelbrecht, Dr Claus Kohnlein, Dr Samantha Bailey, MD, Dr Stefano Scoglio, MD p 166-167

88 Dr. William Trebing, Goodbye Germ Theory P 161

89 VIRUS MANIA: Avian Flu (H5N1), Cervical Cancer (HPV), SARS, BSE, Hepatitis C, AIDS, Polio…How the Medical Industry Continually Invents Epidemics, Making Billion-Dollar Profits at Our Expense by Torsten Engelbrecht, Dr Claus Kohnlein, Dr Samantha Bailey, MD, Dr Stefano Scoglio, MD p 159

90 www.Rumble.com Scoundrel Weapon Information Distribution Channel June 24, 2021

91 The Truth About Contagion by Thomas S. Cowan, MD and Sally Fallon Morell p 51

92 The Truth About Contagion by Thomas S. Cowan, MD and Sally Fallon Morell p 51

93 Dr. Wu Zunyou, MD, PhD, is the Chief Epidemiologist of Chinese Center for Disease Control and Prevention, and an Adjunct Professor of Epidemiology at University of California at Los Angeles.

94 andrewkaufmanmd.com

95   The Real Anthony Fauci" Bill Gates, Big Pharma, and the Global War on Democracy and Public Health by Robert F. Kennedy, Jr. p 446

96   The Real Anthony Fauci" Bill Gates, Big Pharma, and the Global War on Democracy and Public Health by Robert F. Kennedy, Jr. pp 126

97   Kary Mullis Interview https://www.youtube.com/watch?v=RE0e7gj6x20

98   There's more to Vaccination than the Shot by Sharon Kimmelman

99   PF Colliers Encyclopedia, 1983

100 Good-bye Germ Theory, William Trebing

101 Good-bye Germ Theory, William Trebing

102 Turtles All The Way Down – Vaccine Science and Myth p 37

103 ibid. p 52

104 ibid. p 53

105 ibid. p 52

106 ibid. p 57

107 ibid. p 58

108 ibid. p 64, 65

109 ibid. p 70

110 ibid. p 75

111 ibid. p 82

112 ibid. p 237

113 ibid. p 239

114 "The Real Anthony Fauci" Bill Gates, Big Pharma, and the Global War on Democracy and Public Health by Robert F. Kennedy, Jr.

115 Five Biological Laws of Nature – 5BN – Scientific Chart of German New Medicine by Dr. med. Mag. Theol. Ryke Geerd Hamer; 5 Biological Laws and Dr. Hamer's New Medicine by Andrea Taddei

116 Five Biological Laws of Nature – 5BN – Scientific Chart of German New Medicine by Dr. med. Mag. Theol. Ryke Geerd Hamer p 5

117 Five Biological Laws of Nature – 5BN – Scientific Chart of German New Medicine by Dr. med. Mag. Theol. Ryke Geerd Hamer; 5 Biological Laws and Dr. Hamer's New Medicine by Andrea Taddei

118 www.Learninggnm.com

119 ibid.

120 ibid.

121 ibid.

www.ingramcontent.com/pod-product-compliance
Lightning Source LLC
Chambersburg PA
CBHW062217270326
41930CB00009B/1762